# New Wars and Old Plagues

Katherine Hirschfeld • Kirsten de Beurs
Brad Brayfield • Ani Melkonyan-Gottschalk

# New Wars and Old Plagues

## Armed Conflict, Environmental Change and Resurgent Malaria in the Southern Caucasus

palgrave
macmillan

Katherine Hirschfeld
Department of Anthropology
University of Oklahoma
Norman, OK, USA

Brad Brayfield
Department of Anthropology
University of Oklahoma
Norman, OK, USA

Kirsten de Beurs
Laboratory of Geo-information
Science and Remote Sensing
Wageningen University and Research
Wageningen, The Netherlands

Ani Melkonyan-Gottschalk
ZLV, Joint Centre Urban
Systems, Rm 912
University of Duisburg-Essen
Duisburg, Nordrhein-Westfalen
Germany

ISBN 978-3-031-31142-0 ISBN 978-3-031-31143-7 (eBook)
https://doi.org/10.1007/978-3-031-31143-7



This Palgrave Macmillan imprint is published by the registered company Springer Nature Switzerland AG.
The registered company address is: Gewerbestrasse 11, 6330 Cham, Switzerland

*This book is dedicated to Xander and Maryn, who went through the most difficult things a child could experience and somehow made their parents stronger. We will forever admire your strength, perseverance and determination.*

# Acknowledgments

This book is a collaborative project and we have many people to thank for sharing their time, recollections and resources with us. We are grateful to Dr. Scott McNabb of the Centers for Disease Control for talking with us about his experiences as an Epidemiology Intelligence Service officer in Armenia. Thomas Goltz provided maps, photos and insights from his time as a journalist embedded in Azerbaijan in the 1990s. All the archivists at the National Archives facility in College Park, Maryland were incredibly helpful locating relevant record collections.

During our first site visit to Armenia in 2018 members of our research group were graciously received by a number of research scientists. These included Dr. Levon Vardanyan and Dr. Hamlet Melkonyan of the Hydrometerological Service, Dr. Diana Harutyunyan from the Ministry of Nature Protection, Dr. Hovik Sayadyan from the UNDP office, Dr. Artak Pilpoyan of Yerevan State University and Dr. Ara Keshishyan from the Ministry of Health. Dr. David Pipoyan from the Ecocenter at the National Academy of Sciences provided us with information about land use and land cover monitoring in Armenia. Dr. Gurgen Yeghiazaryan of the Department of Hydrotechnology and Dr. Alen Amirkhanyan from the American University in Armenia shared very useful irrigation maps and land cover maps. Dr. Abraham Ghazaryan showed us some of the accomplishments of the Scientific Center of Agriculture and Plant Protection and the Experimental Farm of Echmiadzin. We are also thankful to Dr. Caroline Wegner of the German International Cooperation project for sharing information about biodiversity in the Caucasus.

We would also like to thank several research groups and individuals for providing data and extending their kindness during our second field visit to Armenia in 2022. These included Dr. Lusine Paronyan and her staff at the National Center for Disease Control and Prevention within the Ministry of Health. A special thank you goes to Dr. Ara Keshishyan for his invaluable discussions on historical malaria and control efforts within Armenia. Nune Asatryan and her staff at the United Nations International Organization for Migration in Yerevan for providing a summary of the migration and refugee status and their efforts during the fall 2020 war. We are also thankful to George Comai for insightful suggestions following our panel presentation at the Association for the Study of Nationalities conference in 2021. Braden Owsley helped navigate rural villages during our fieldwork in Armenia and contributed his excellent technical skills for the remote sensing work, along with James Worden and Masha Jami.

Volker Radeloff and Johanna Buchner generously shared data and insights on our ASN conference panel in 2021.

This research would not have been possible without the outstanding administrative support provided by Ms. Emalee Lemke in the Department of Geography and Environmental Sustainability and Ms. Misty Wilson in the Department of Anthropology at the University of Oklahoma. Lastly, we are indebted to all the residents in Armenia who took the time to accompany us during fieldwork.

We attest we have no conflicts of interest related to the preparation of this work.

This research was supported by the NASA: Land-Cover/Land-Use Change project entitled "Land use patterns and political instability as predictors for the re-emergence of malaria in the Caucasus" to Kirsten de Beurs and Katherine Hirschfeld. Project number: 16-LCLUC16-2-0017.

# About the Book

This book began as a collection of papers presented virtually at the May 2021 meetings of the Association for the Study of Nationalities (ASN). The title of our panel was "Landscapes of Ethnicity, Conflict and Environmental Change in the Caucasus." Our papers explored social or environmental dimensions of the Karabakh conflict and we came away from the panel impressed by the unique insights gained from integrating research from social science, natural science and global health. Several audience members shared their appreciation of our multi-disciplinary approach and with that encouragement we began to develop our conference papers into a collaborative book manuscript. We are very grateful to Ms. Elizabeth Graber and the editorial staff at Palgrave Macmillan for their support for this project.

The overall goal of this work is to explore how ethnic conflict reshaped the social and environmental landscape and created a lasting population health crisis in the southern Caucasus following the collapse of the Soviet Union. In 1988 a war between Armenia and Azerbaijan began over the contested Karabakh region, and violence intensified until a cease fire agreement in 1994. The conflict reignited in December 2020 and tensions remain high in the region. While the Karabakh conflict itself has been the subject of a number of academic analyses, existing works have focused primarily on ethnic violence and the complex international relations of the immediate post-Soviet period. Environmental damage and population health crises have not received comparable attention in academic literature. This oversight is important because (as a number of classic works in disease ecology have demonstrated) infectious disease outbreaks associated with warfare often kill more people than the armed conflicts themselves. Warfare itself has also changed dramatically since the collapse of the USSR, and the Karabakh conflict provides an informative case study of the way these "New Wars" transform the natural and social environment to facilitate outbreaks of preventable disease. We believe this extended case study will be useful to researchers from a variety of academic disciplines, including geography, conflict studies, disease ecology, medical anthropology, global health and public health. It also reveals the fragility of twentieth-century malaria control in temperate regions and will assist in predictive modeling for future outbreaks.

# Contents

# About the Authors

**Kirsten de Beurs** is Professor and Chair in the Laboratory of Geo-information Science and Remote Sensing at Wageningen University in the Netherlands. She obtained a PhD in Natural Resource Sciences and is interested in the analysis of earth observation data related to terrestrial ecosystems. She has authored over 100 articles and book chapters focused on the analysis of land cover and land use changes and their impacts using remotely sensed data.

**Brad Brayfield** is a PhD candidate in the Department of Anthropology at the University of Oklahoma. His dissertation research explores human mobility and forced migration in relation to Anthropocene environmental change and non-state warfare.

**Katherine Hirschfeld** is a Professor in the Department of Anthropology at the University of Oklahoma. She is a medical anthropologist interested in political instability, armed conflict and disease ecology. Her previous books include *Gangster-States: Organized Crime, Kleptocracy and Political Collapse*, published by Palgrave Macmillan in 2015, and *Health, Politics and Revolution in Cuba since 1898*, published by Transaction Press in 2007.

**Ani Melkonyan-Gottschalk** is Executive Director of the Centre for Logistics and Traffic, University of Duisburg-Essen in Germany. Prof. Melkonyan-Gottschalk has been active in research and teaching in fundamental areas of sustainable economies and transformation frameworks toward sustainable and smart governance for more than 13 years. Prof. Melkonyan-Gottschalk has expertise in sustainable and smart urban regions, sustainable supply chain management, holistic urban mobility and logistics systems, digital and innovative business ecosystems and sustainable inclusive governance models.

# Abbreviations

| | |
|---|---|
| ACAPS | Assessment Capacities Project |
| AO | Autonomous Oblast |
| ASN | Association for the Study of Nationalities |
| ASSR | Autonomous Soviet Socialist Republic |
| CDC | Centers for Disease Control |
| DDT | Dichlorodiphenyltrichloroethane |
| EIS | Epidemiology Intelligence Service |
| GAP | Southeastern Anatolia Irrigation Project |
| IDP | Internally Displaced Persons |
| IDMC | International Displacement Monitoring Center |
| IOM | United Nations International Organization of Migration |
| IPCC | Inter Governmental Panel on Climate Change |
| NKAO | Nagorno-Karabakh Administrative Oblast |
| NGK | Nagorno-Karabakh |
| OSCE | Organization for Security and Cooperation in Europe |
| PHEIC | Public Health Emergency of International Concern |
| PR-2020 | Post 2020 Boundary Reconfiguration of Nagorno-Karabakh |
| PRIO | Peace Resolution Institute Oslo |
| PROBA-V | Project for On Board Autonomy |
| SARS-CoV-2 | SARS Corona Virus 2 |
| SSR | Soviet Socialist Republic |
| TWI | Topographic Wetness Index |
| UNECE | United Nations Economic Commission for Europe |
| UNHCR | United Nations High Commissioner for Refugees |

| | |
|---|---|
| USAID | United States Agency for International Development |
| USSR | Union of Soviet Socialist Republics (Soviet Union) |
| WHO | World Health Organization |

# List of Figures

CHAPTER 1

# Introduction

**Abstract** This chapter provides an overview of the Karabakh conflict and describes its importance for understanding population health crises that emerge from "New Wars." The most intense phase of fighting in Karabakh coincided with the region's first epidemic of *Plasmodium vivax* malaria since the 1950s. While the malaria epidemic was documented in public health scholarship, the chaotic environment of the conflict meant that very little investigation was done into the re-emergence of this ancestral vector borne disease after decades of successful control. This chapter includes a discussion of the usefulness of combining qualitative historical work with remote sensing data to reconstruct the social and environmental changes that took place in and around the conflict zone. We also discuss the significance of the work and the need for updated models to explain the growing prevalence of "New Wars" and their relationship to global health risks.

**Keywords** Karabakh • Caucasus • Malaria • Remote sensing

In the early decades of the twentieth century, the Soviet Union consistently enchanted foreign visitors with its plans for radical transformation of humankind. Belief in the power of Soviet science to end suffering and disease was a consistent theme in the memoirs of idealistic travelers (Hollander 1998). In 1928 one enthusiastic visitor predicted the combined wisdom of Lenin and Pasteur would soon eradicate all hunger and


K. Hirschfeld et al., *New Wars and Old Plagues*,
https://doi.org/10.1007/978-3-031-31143-7_1

disease. "The future!" he exclaimed, "is our victory … the victory of communism signifies the salvation of humanity" (Carbo 1928: 70).

Over one hundred years later, it is understood that the Soviet Union did not bring about the salvation of humanity or the perfection of human health. Instead, the USSR collapsed into conflict-ridden rubble after decades of economic stagnation and authoritarian repression. But there are still a number of important lessons to be found between the hopeful beginnings and violent ends of the Soviet experiment. Once excavated these lessons have the potential to help contemporary researchers understand the kinds of health and humanitarian crises that emerge in the aftermath of armed conflicts.

This book presents an extended case study of one ethnic conflict and associated epidemiological crises from the southern Caucasus. The Karabakh war took place in rugged mountainous territory between Armenia and Azerbaijan. The area is approximately 4800 $km^2$, approximately 1.5 times the size of the US state of Rhode Island (Croissant 1998: 10). The mountainous region is heavily forested while the valleys are generally occupied by croplands, vineyards and orchards (see Fig. 1.1 for a detailed outline map of the conflict area).

Hostilities began in 1987 and despite several peace accords, tensions remain high in the region. This makes the Karabakh conflict the most prolonged territorial dispute in post-Soviet Eurasia. The most intense phase of fighting lasted from 1988–1994. New hostilities have broken out repeatedly since that time, with major escalation in 2020 and periodic outbreaks of violence through 2022.

As Mary Kaldor described, the Karabakh conflict represents a new kind of warfare that is different from the nation-state wars that defined the early decades of the twentieth century. "New Wars," (as she termed them) are typically waged between non-state or sub-state actors, involve ethnic or religious violence as well as violence against civilians (2007, 2012). New Wars often have an economic substrate in the informal economy with combatants financing their insurgencies in ways that can intersect with international organized crime. "New Wars," Kaldor concludes, "are associated with state weakness, extremist identity politics and transnational criminality" (2012: 8). A growing number of conflicts fit this pattern and their expansion coincides with the decline of twentieth-century institutions of nation-state governance in many parts of the world (Bunker 2015; Trabulsi 2015; Gilman 2014).

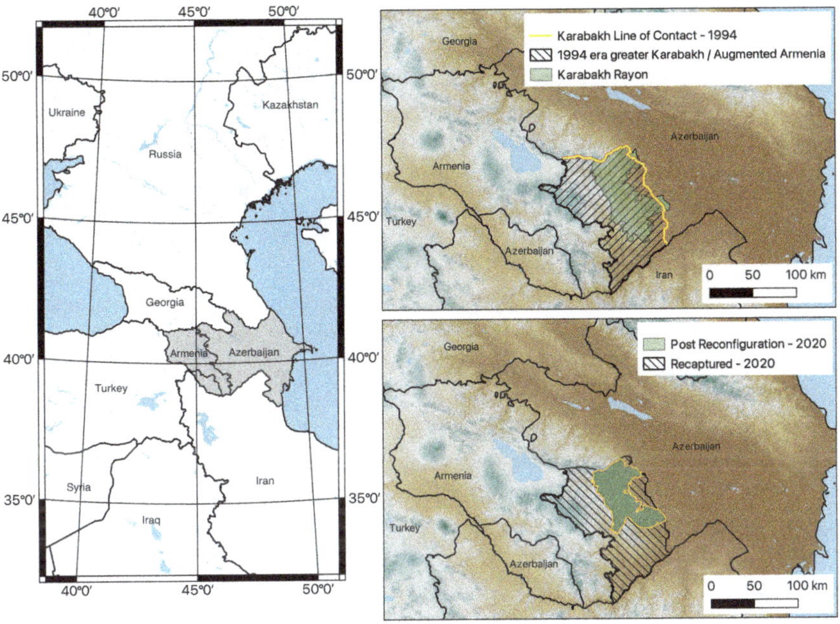


**Fig. 1.1** Outline map of conflict area. The Nagorno-Karabakh line of contact was downloaded from the website of the Armenian Ministry of Foreign Affairs (digitized on GitHub by https://github.com/mkudamatsu/data_karabakh-map). The country borders and the original Nagorno-Karabakh boundary are from the ESRI country and disputed boundaries databases. We have conflated the shapefiles of the line of contact to the country and Nagorno-Karabakh delineation

Kaldor and other researchers have described how non-state actors often take on informal governance functions in territories fragmented by New War conflicts, and these activities can become quite profitable over time (Kaldor 2007; Mandic 2021). This creates an array of perverse incentives for prolonged conflict and instability as war-making can become more lucrative than peace-making (Andreas 2010). For these and other reasons, state-building in the aftermath of New Wars can be difficult and vulnerable to failure.

Because New Wars involve indiscriminate attacks on civilians and social institutions (including schools and health care facilities), they can be challenging for researchers to study in real time. Quantitative survey research can be difficult in an environment with limited infrastructure. Qualitative information from conflict zones is fragmented and security risks to researchers can be high. After his extensive work on the Chechen conflict of the 1990s, for instance, anthropologist Valery Tishkov concluded that conventional ethnographic methods are ineffective in New War environments, "…Information obtained under such conditions is full of slogans, manifestos and intense emotions absent in a calmer climate. Informants may be in such an agitated state that one can record only the background noise of an imposed reality that is often mistaken for 'hard reality'" (2004: 4).

For these and other reasons we developed a set of spatially and temporally distanced methods to undertake a retrospective analysis of the Karabakh conflict. Qualitative historical and anthropological methods were combined with quantitative geospatial research and census data to reconstruct key elements of the conflict and explore its effects on the natural environment. The goal was to better understand the relationship between New Wars, environmental change and population health crises. These methods are detailed in Appendix A.

During the most intense phase of the Karabakh conflict in the 1990s, there was an epidemic of *Plasmodium vivax* (*P. vivax*) malaria in Armenia and Azerbaijan. This was the first recorded outbreak of this ancestral vector borne disease in the Caucasus since malaria was declared eradicated by Soviet authorities in the 1960s. Malaria is one of humanity's most persistent pathogens (Carter and Mendis 2002; Packard 2007; Shah 2010). There are several varieties of malaria, with *P. vivax* best adapted to transmission in northern latitudes (White 2011). The disease was once endemic in the USSR, and devastating epidemics were common in the river valleys of the southern Caucasus in the early years of the twentieth century (Hackett 1937; Johnson 1988; League of Nations 1934; Packard 2017). Soviet authorities undertook aggressive eradication campaigns after World War I, but did not succeed in fully controlling the disease for many decades (Johnson 1988).

The reappearance of malaria in the Caucasus during the conflict period of the 1990s indicates that a number of environmental changes took place in a short period of time to make the region newly hospitable to the anopheles mosquito vector. These changes escaped the attention of journalists and scholars embedded in the conflict, who were naturally more focused on the humanitarian crises, territorial instability and fragile political coalitions of the newly independent Caucasus republics.[1] Once malaria was detected in Armenia a team of epidemiologists from the Centers for

Disease Control in Atlanta was dispatched to work with Armenian health authorities to control the outbreak (Centers for Disease Control 1998). But these efforts were primarily focused on the basic work of identifying cases and reducing transmission in a time of extreme crisis. Public health professionals in Armenia did not have an opportunity to explore the larger social or environmental changes that allowed the disease to return to the region after such a prolonged absence.

The Karabakh conflict also merits renewed attention for geopolitical reasons. As Michael Croissant wrote in 1998, "Not only is the Armenia-Azerbaijan conflict one of the bloodiest and most intractable clashes to emerge from the breakup of the Soviet empire, but it is also the only remaining post-Soviet conflict that poses a potentially explosive threat to peace and security on a regional—as opposed to a local—scale" (p. xi). In other words, the southern Caucasus region is located at the intersection of alliances and rivalries between a number of regional powers including Russia, Iran and Turkey. Ongoing tensions in the region signify the potential for a much larger conflict to emerge in the future (Cicero 2020; Crisis Group 2022a, 2022b, 2022c).

What will happen in the Caucasus if widespread instability and armed conflict return to the region? Unfortunately, our research suggests the potential for synergistic outbreaks of old and new pathogens. In addition to malaria, the Karabakh conflict triggered resurgent epidemics of tuberculosis, measles, diphtheria and typhoid fever (Dudwick 1997; Grigorian 1992; Shapiro 1993). Since that time, there have been multiple PHEICs (Public Health Emergencies of International Concern) as global environmental instability, climate change and urbanization continue to accelerate the evolution and spread of new diseases (Hotez 2009; Shah 2016). These developments suggest that any future conflict could easily result in higher mortality from infectious disease than from combat itself (Price-Smith 2008).

Even without formal hostilities, the next few decades are likely to see accelerating waves of human migration and global health risks due to climate change. These population flows will increase risks of other tropical diseases emerging or re-emerging in northern latitudes (Hotez 2016). The United Nations and the World Health Organization recognize human mobility's relationship to conflict, the changing climate and global health. They urge the development of a comprehensive migrant health agenda that accounts for both long term and acute human mobility (WHO 2018; IDMC 2020).

Remote sensing—the use of satellite images to understand land cover and land use changes—and other distanced methods offer indirect ways to assess the impact of New War conflicts on the environment and vulnerable human populations. Changes in land use, for instance, are recognized as one of the most important variables in the emergence of novel pandemic pathogens (Keesing et al. 2010). Several researchers have also developed techniques for using satellite data to track changes in mosquito habitat, and this work has been usefully applied to assess risks of dengue fever, malaria and West Nile Virus (Anno et al. 2019; Chuang and Wimberly 2012; McMahon et al. 2021; Wimberly et al. 2021). Remote sensing data has also been used to measure rates of abandoned cropland in Eastern Europe and Russia—a key variable in the formation of new mosquito habitat (de Beurs et al. 2016; de Beurs and Ioffe 2014; Griffiths et al. 2014; Lioubimtseva et al. 2013; Meyfroidt et al. 2016; Prishchepov et al. 2017) as well as in Central Asia (de Beurs and Henebry 2004; de Beurs et al. 2018; Horion et al. 2016; Prishchepov et al. 2017). Fewer studies have been focused on the Caucasus (Buchner et al. 2020; Melkonyan 2014, 2015), but they reveal significant forest cover changes as a result of the first Karabakh conflict (Baumann et al. 2015; Buchner et al. 2020).

When combined with qualitative historical and anthropological research, remote sensing data have the potential to create an "expanded epidemiology" to improve analysis of population health crises in New War conflict zones or other regions that are difficult for researchers to access. This extended case study method situates anomalous disease outbreaks deeper in time, across broader geographies, and within more richly contextualized environmental and social histories than conventional work in public health. Remote sensing also allows environmental instability to be rendered visually, in the form of maps that reveal changes in cropland, population flows, water resources and forest cover.

This small book seeks to integrate these environmental, epidemiological and social analyses together in a transdisciplinary framework that we hope will be useful for other researchers interested in the relationship between armed conflict, environmental change and population health. The work is organized into five chapters. Chapter 2 presents a qualitative historical overview of the Caucasus region during the Soviet and post-Soviet conflict periods, including its time as a malaria hotspot in the early twentieth century. One of the goals of this chapter is to remind contemporary audiences that controlling *P. vivax* required decades of authoritarian social and environmental engineering across broad swaths of territory in the USSR and Europe (Hackett 1937; Johnson 1988; Shah 2010). Much of this history has been forgotten, and malaria is typically categorized as a tropical disease by contemporary global health scholars (Packard 2017). This errant classification may blind contemporary researchers to the vulnerability of Russia and the Caucasus republics to new outbreaks of *P. vivax*.

Chapter 2 also connects the institutional and ideological decay of formal Soviet institutions—including the institutions of centralized economic planning—to the emergence of an extensive kin-based informal economy in the late Soviet period. As several scholars have described, the informal economy in the Soviet Union functioned as a space of anti-Soviet resistance while also preserving an array of pre-Soviet institutions and regional cultural practices (de Waal 2013; Dudwick 1997; King 2008; Koehler and Zurcher 2003a; Zurcher 2007). Over time, these informal institutions configured "a parallel social order" that often superseded the official institutions of the formal Soviet system, which remained paralyzed by inefficiency and bureaucratic inertia (Koehler and Zurcher 2003b: 150). Once the formal Soviet system collapsed, these informal systems quickly formalized in ways that intensified ethnic and clan-based divisions. Tensions were especially acute in Karabakh due to its status as an Armenian enclave located within the larger political geography of Soviet Azerbaijan.

Chapter 3 presents a compressed historical overview of the first Karabakh conflict period from 1988 until the cease fire agreement in 1994. When the USSR collapsed in 1991 the Karabakh conflict expanded into formal warfare between neighboring states. Both sides were armed with sophisticated Soviet weaponry (Goltz 1998). As Mary Kaldor described, "The war involved fractions of the Soviet army, volunteer militias and paramilitary groups, and criminal gangs as well as the newly established armies of Azerbaijan, Karabakh and Armenia" (2007: 159). In a few short years, there were massive population displacements and repeated cycles of ethnic violence and forced migration. A detailed chronology of the conflict is provided in Appendix B.

Chapter 4 explores the health and humanitarian crises generated by the Karabakh conflict. The UN International Organization of Migration (IOM), a leading inter-governmental organization on migration, stresses the increasing importance of human migration and its role as a social determinant of health (WHO 2018). It is estimated that approximately one million people were displaced from Karabakh and neighboring rayons because of conflict, with the vast majority being Azerbaijani (UNHCR Report 2009). Many of these displaced persons settled in Baku and other regional centers, but hundreds of thousands were also placed in UNHCR camps in regions east of NK and in lowland areas of Azerbaijan.

In addition to malaria, Armenia and other war-torn countries in the Caucasus suffered a number of epidemics of preventable diseases during and after the conflict period in the 1990s, along with prolonged food and energy shortages. Most of the disease outbreaks were controlled with vaccination campaigns and the restoration of public health and municipal services. Malaria, however, is a complex vector-borne disease that cannot be understood without a broader environmental analysis that includes water systems, population mobility and land use patterns.

Overall our remote sensing data reveals the Karabakh conflict had lasting environmental impacts on forests, towns, farmsteads and agricultural production. Logging and forest fires were widespread and many formerly productive croplands fell into a semi-permanent state of abandonment after the 1994 peace accord. Failure to maintain irrigation systems created expansive new mosquito habitat. Even today much of the region remains underpopulated due to ongoing tensions and low intensity conflict.

The Karabakh conflict erupted again in the fall of 2020 with intense fighting over six weeks. Thousands of people were killed and many more displaced. Russia brokered a cease fire agreement that led to an uneasy peace, followed by periodic outbursts of violence. The 2020 peace plan included significant territorial reconfiguration, with areas controlled by Armenia since the 1990s scheduled to be returned to Azerbaijan. In the fall of 2022 protests took place in Armenia against the transfer of these lands. These events are detailed in Chap. 5, which includes a longitudinal analysis of environmental change in the Karabakh region due to years of intermittent violence coupled with multiple rounds of forced migration and resettlement.

In his history of the Karabakh conflict, Thomas de Waal states, "It will take many years for a full picture of what happened in Armenia and Azerbaijan after 1988 to be assembled" (2013: ix). This work attempts to add several new pieces to this complex picture by incorporating information from above and below the human level of perception. Remote sensing data allows us to explore macro level environmental changes associated with the conflict. Incorporating historical and epidemiological research allows us to explore how the conflict facilitated the invasion of microscopic pathogens into vulnerable human bodies.

Overall this work reveals the benefit of integrating material from multiple fields of study to address the connections between armed conflict, environmental change and population health. Specifically, we believe New War conflicts are likely to interact synergistically with climate change in the coming years to generate epidemics of infectious and vector borne diseases that were successfully controlled during the twentieth century. The decline of nation-state governance and erosion of public health prevention measures in many places over the past two decades could easily amplify local outbreaks into regional or global health hazards (Hirschfeld 2019).

If history is any guide the reappearance of these ancestral diseases in the Caucasus could also play a major role in determining the outcome of future conflicts. In analyzing the role of malaria infection among troops in World War I, for instance, malariologist L.W. Hackett described British, French and German armies as completely incapacitated by the disease in 1916, "We had the spectacle of three fine armies, backed by the most powerful nations of Europe and equipped regardless of expense with every modern appointment, virtually paralyzed [by malaria] before they could strike a blow" (1937: 2). For these reasons we believe widespread return of malaria to the Caucasus or Europe could accelerate what some social scientists have termed the "third epidemiological transition." This refers to a lasting change in overall population mortality from non-infectious to infectious diseases, even in countries that have successfully achieved a "modern" health and mortality profile for many decades (Barrett and Armelagos 2014).

## Note

1. There are several excellent accounts of the Karabakh conflict written by journalists. Two of the best are *Azerbaijan Diary* by Thomas Goltz and *Black Garden* by Thomas de Waal. Our research group had an opportunity to speak with Mr. Goltz about his experiences during the war, and he indicated he had no awareness of the malaria outbreak. Various professionals we spoke with during our sites visits also had little or no awareness that malaria had returned to Armenia in the 1990s.

## References

Andreas, Peter. 2010. *Blue Helmets and Black Markets: The Business of Survival in the Siege of Sarajevo*. Ithaca: Cornell University Press.

Anno, Sumiko, Takeshi Hara, Hiroki Kai, Ming-An Lee, Yi Chang, Kei Oyoshi, Yousel Mizukami, and Takeo Tadono. 2019. Spatiotemporal Dengue Fever Hotspots Associated with Climatic Factors in Taiwan Including Outbreak Predictions Based on Machine-Learning. *Geospatial Health* 14(2). https://geospatialhealth.net/index.php/gh/article/view/771. Accessed 22 August 2022.

Barrett, Ron, and George Armelagos. 2014. *An Unnatural History of Emerging Infections*. Oxford: Oxford University Press.

Baumann, Matthias, Volker Radeloff, Vahagn Avedian, and Tobias Kuemmerle. 2015. Land Use Change in the Caucasus During and After the Nagorno-Karabakh Conflict. *Regional Environmental Change* 15 (8): 1703–1716.

Buchner, Johanna, He Yin, David Frantz, Tobias Kuemmerle, Elshad Askerov, Tamar Bakuradze, Benjamin Bleyhl, Nodar Elizbarashvili, Anna Komarova, Katarzyna E. Lewińska, Afag Rizayeva, Hovik Sayadyan, Bin Tank, Garegin Tepanosyan, Nugzar Zazanashvilie, and Volker C. Radeloff. 2020. Land-Cover Change in the Caucasus Mountains since 1987 Based on the Topographic Correction of Multi-temporal Landsat Composites. *Remote Sensing of Environment* 248: 111967.

Bunker, Robert. 2015. Forward: Violent Entrepreneurs and Techno Warlords: All Edge. In *Warlords, Inc., Black Markets, Broken States and the Rise of the Warlord Entrepreneur*, ed. Noah Raford and Andrew Trabulsi, 13–26. Berkeley: North Atlantic Books.

Carbo, Sergio. 1928. *Un Viaje a La Rusia Roja*. La Habana: Ediciones Revista Avance.

Carter, Richard, and Kamini N. Mendis. 2002. Evolutionary and Historical Aspects of the Burden of Malaria. *Clinical Microbiology Reviews* 15 (4): 564–594.

Centers for Disease Control (CDC). 1998. Epidemic Malaria Transmission in Armenia, 1997. *Morbidity and Mortality Weekly Report* 47 (25): 526–528. https://www.cdc.gov/mmwr/preview/mmwrhtml/00053695.htm. Accessed 4 Sept. 2020.

Chuang, Ting-Wu, and Michael Wimberly. 2012. Remote Sensing of Climatic Anomalies and West Nile Virus Incidence in the Northern Great Plains of the United States. *PLOS One* 7 (10): e46882. https://pubmed.ncbi.nlm.nih.gov/23071656. Accessed 22 August 2022.

Cicero, Michael. 2020. Escalation and Regional Risks in a New Karabakh War. https://www.mei.edu/publications/escalation-and-regional-risks-new-karabakh-war. Accessed 22 September 2022.

Crisis Group 2022a. Warding Off Renewed War in Nagorno-Karabakh. https://www.crisisgroup.org/europe-central-asia/caucasus/nagorno-karabakh-conflict/warding-renewed-war-nagorno-karabakh. Accessed 22 September 2022.

———. 2022b. The Nagorno-Karabakh Conflict: A Visual Explainer. https://www.crisisgroup.org/content/nagorno-karabakh-conflict-visual-explainer. Accessed 29 October 2022.

———. 2022c. Upholding the Ceasefire between Azerbaijan and Armenia. September 28. https://www.crisisgroup.org/europe-central-asia/caucasus/armenia-azerbaijannagorno-karabakh-conflict/upholding-ceasefire. Accessed 29 October 2022.

Croissant, Michael. 1998. *The Armenia-Azerbaijan Conflict: Causes and Implications*. Westport, CT: Praeger.

de Beurs, Kirsten M., and Geoffrey M. Henebry. 2004. Land Surface Phenology, Climatic Variation, and Institutional Change: Analyzing Agricultural Land Cover Change in Kazakhstan. *Remote Sensing of Environment* 89. https://doi.org/10.1016/j.rse.2003.11.006.

de Beurs, Kirsten M., and Grigory Ioffe. 2014. Use of Landsat and MODIS Data to Remotely Estimate Russia's Sown Area. *Journal of Land Use Science* 9. https://doi.org/10.1080/1747423X.2013.798038.

de Beurs, Kirsten, Grigory Ioffe, Tatyana Nefedova, and Geoffrey Henebry. 2016. Land Change in European Russia: 1982–2011. In *Land-Cover and Land-Use Changes in Eastern Europe after the Collapse of the Soviet Union in 1991*, ed. Garik Gutman and Volker Radeloff. Switzerland: Springer International Publishing AG. https://doi.org/10.1007/978-3-319-42638-9_10.

de Beurs, Kirsten M., Geoffrey M. Henebry, Braden C. Owsley, and Irina N. Sokolik. 2018. Large Scale Climate Oscillation Impacts on Temperature, Precipitation and Land Surface Phenology in Central Asian. *Environmental Research Letters* 13: 065018. https://doi.org/10.1088/1748-9326/aac4d0.

de Waal, Thomas. 2013. *Black Garden: Armenia and Azerbaijan Through Peace and War*. New York: New York University Press.

Dudwick, Nora. 1997. Political Transformation in Post-communist Armenia: Images and Realities. In *Conflict, Cleavage and Change in Central Asia and the Caucasus*, ed. Karen Dawisha and Bruce Parrott, 69–109. Cambridge: Cambridge University Press.

Gilman, Nils. 2014. The Twin Insurgency. *The American Interest*. https://www.the-americaninterest.com/2014/06/15/the-twin-insurgency/. Accessed 12 September 2022.

Goltz, Thomas. 1998. *Azerbaijan Diary*. Armonk, NY: M.E. Sharpe.

Griffiths, Patrick, Tobias Kuemmerle, Matthias Baumann, Volker C. Radeloff, Ioan V. Abrudan, Juraj Lieskovsky, Catalina Munteanu, Katarzyna Ostapowicz, and Patrick Hostert. 2014. Forest Disturbances, Forest Recovery, and Changes in Forest Types Across the Carpathian Ecoregion from 1985 to 2010 Based on Landsat Image Composites. *Remote Sensing of Environment* 151: 72–88.

Grigorian, Stella. 1992. *Fax Letter to Aryeh Cooperstock, Henryka Manes and Gabrielle Brook*. January 29. Retrieved from RG 0268 Records of the United States Agency for International Development, National Archives and Records Administration, College Park, Maryland.

Hackett, Lewis W. 1937. *Malaria in Europe: An Ecological Survey.* London: Oxford University Press.

Hirschfeld, Katherine. 2019. Microbial Insurgency: Theorizing Global Health in the Anthropocene. *Anthropocene Review* 7 (1): 3–18. https://journals.sagepub.com/eprint/S9TCTCM6GB8INSS9TQXP/full. Accessed 24 August 2022.

Hollander, Paul. 1998. *Political Pilgrims: Western Intellectuals in Search of the Good Society.* New Brunswick, NJ: Transaction Press.

Horion, Stéphanie, Alexander V. Prishchepov, Jan Verbesselt, Kirsten de Beurs, Torbern Tagesson, and Rasmus Fensholt. 2016. Revealing Turning Points in Ecosystem Functioning over the Northern Eurasian Agricultural Frontier. *Global Change Biology* 22. https://doi.org/10.1111/gcb.13267.

Hotez, Peter. 2009. Waging Peace Through Neglected Tropical Disease Control. *PLOS Neglected Tropical Disease Control* 3 (1): e346. https://doi.org/10.1371/journal.pntd.0000346. Accessed 16 September 2022.

———. 2016. *Blue Marble Health: An Innovative Plan to Fight Diseases of the poor Amid Wealth.* Baltimore, Maryland: Johns Hopkins University Press.

Internal Displacement Monitoring Centre (IDMC). 2020. Global Report on Internal Displacement. https://www.internal-displacement.org/global-report/grid2020/. Accessed 30 October 2022.

Johnson, Richard. 1988. *Malaria and Malaria Control in the USSR*, 1917–1941. PhD thesis, Georgetown University Department of History.

Kaldor, Mary. 2007. Oil and Conflict: The Case of Nagorno-Karabakh. In *Oil Wars*, ed. Mary Kaldor, Terry Lynn Karl, and Yahia Said, 157–182. London: Pluto Press.

———. 2012. *Old and New Wars.* Malden, MA: Polity Press.

Keesing, Felicia, Lisa K. Belden, Peter Daszak, Andrew Dobson, C. Drew Harvell, Robert D. Holt, Peter Hudson, Anna Jolles, Kate E. Jones, Charles E. Mitchell, Samuel S. Myers, Tiffany Bogich, and Richard S. Ostfeld. 2010. Impacts of Biodiversity on the Emergence and Transmission of Infectious Diseases. *Nature*, 468 (7324): 647–652. https://www.ncbi.nlm.nih.gov/pmc/articles/PMC7094913/. Accessed 22 August 2022.

King, Charles. 2008. *The Ghost of Freedom: A History of the Caucasus.* Oxford: Oxford University Press.

Koehler, Jan, and Christoph Zurcher. 2003a. Introduction. In *Potentials of Disorder: New Approaches to Conflict Analysis*, ed. Jan Koehler and Christoph Zurcher, 1–12. Manchester: Manchester University Press.

———. 2003b. The Art of Losing the State: Weak Empire to Weak Nation-State Around Nagorno-Karabakh. In *Potentials of Disorder: New Approaches to Conflict Analysis*, ed. Jan Koehler and Christoph Zurcher, 145–173. Manchester: Manchester University Press.

League of Nations. 1934. *Ten Years of Activity of the Malaria Commission.* Retrieved from RG 90 Records of the United States Public Health Service. National Archives and Records Administration, College Park, Maryland July 2019.

Lioubimtseva, Elena, Kirsten M. de Beurs, and Geoffrey M. Henebry. 2013. Grain Production Trends in Russia, Ukraine, and Kazakhstan in the Context of the Global Climate Variability and Change. In *Climate Change and Water Resources*, The Handbook of Environmental Chemistry, Book 25, ed. Tamim Younos and Caitlin A. Grady. Berlin: Springer Verlag.

Mandic, Danilo. 2021. *Gangsters and Other Statesmen*. Princeton: Princeton University Press.

McMahon, Andrea, Abere Mihretie, Adem A. Ahmed, Mastewal Lake, Worku Awoke, and Michael C. Wimberly. 2021. Remote Sensing of Environmental Risk Factors for Malaria in Different Geographic Contexts. *International Journal of Health Geographics*, 20(1): 28. https://ij-healthgeographics.biomedcentral.com/articles/10.1186/s12942-021-00282-0. Accessed 22 August 2022.

Melkonyan, Ani. 2014. Environmental and Socio-Economic Vulnerability of Agricultural Sector in Armenia. *Science of the Total Environment*, 488: 333–342.

———. 2015. Climate Change Impact on Water Resources and Crop Production in Armenia. *Agricultural Water Management*. 161: 86–101.

Meyfroidt, Patrick, Florian Schierhorn, Alexander V. Prishchepov, Daniel Müller, and Tobias Kuemmerle. 2016. Drivers, Constraints and Trade-offs Associated with Recultivating Abandoned Cropland in Russia, Ukraine and Kazakhstan. *Global Environmental Change* 37: 1–15.

Packard, Randall. 2007. *The Making of a Tropical Disease: A Short History of Malaria*. Baltimore, MD: Johns Hopkins University Press.

Price-Smith, Andrew T. 2008. *Contagion and Chaos: Disease, Ecology and National Security in the Era of Globalization*. Boston: MIT Press.

Prishchepov, Alexander V., Daniel Müller, Matthias Baumann, Tobias Kuemmerle, Camilo Alcantara, and Volker C. Radeloff. 2017. Underlying Drivers and Spatial Determinants of Post-Soviet Agricultural Land Abandonment in Temperate Eastern Europe. In *Land-Cover and Land-Use Changes in Eastern Europe after the Collapse of the Soviet Union in 1991*, 91–117. Springer.

Russian Ministry of Defence of the Russian Federation: Russian peacekeeping forces in Nagorno-Karabakh. Accessed 2020. https://eng.mil.ru/en/russian_peacekeeping_forces/infographics.htm.

Shah, Sonia. 2010. *The Fever: How Malaria Has Ruled Mankind for 500,000 Years*. New York: Farrar, Strauss and Giroux. Ibooks edition.

———. 2016. *Pandemic: Tracking Contagions from Cholera to Ebola and Beyond*. New York: Sarah Crichton Books.

Shapiro, Margaret. 1993. Armenia's Good Life Lost to Misery and Darkness. *Washington Post*. https://www.washingtonpost.com/archive/politics/1993/01/30/armenias-good-life-lostto-misery-darkness-cold/52d00f30-29bb-4508-9fba-bf543000e8ea/. Accessed 22 September 2022.

Tishkov, Valery. 2004. *Chechnya: Life in a War-Torn Society*. Berkeley: University of California Press.

Trabulsi, Andrew. 2015. Warlords, Inc.—A Portrait. In *Warlords, Inc., Black Markets, Broken States and the Rise of the Warlord Entrepreneur*, ed. Noah Raford and Andrew Trabulsi, 27–46. Berkeley: North Atlantic Books.

UNHCR Report. 2009. *Azerbaijan: Analysis of Gaps in the Protection of Internally Displaced Persons (IDPs)*. UN High Commission for Refugees (UNHCR). https://www.unhcr.org/protection/convention/4bd7edbd9/azerbaijan-analysis-gaps-protection-internally-displaced-persons-idps.html.

White, Nicholas J. 2011. Determinants of Relapse Periodicity in *Plasmodium vivax* Malaria. *Malaria Journal*. https://malariajournal.biomedcentral.com/track/pdf/10.1186/1475-2875-10-297. Accessed 18 June 2020.

Wimberly, Michael, Kirsten M. de Beurs, Tatiana V. Loboda, and William K. Pan. 2021. Satellite Observations and Malaria: New Opportunities for Research and Applications. *Trends in Parasitology* 37 (6): 525–537. https://pubmed.ncbi.nlm.nih.gov/33775559/. Accessed 22 August 2022.

World Health Organization (WHO). 2018. Report on the Health of Refugees and Migrants in the WHO European Region. No PUBLIC HEALTH without REFUGEE and MIGRANT HEALTH. WHO Regional Office for Europe. Copenhagen, Denmark. https://www.who.int/publications/i/item/9789240054462. Accessed 30 October 2022.

Zurcher, Christoph. 2007. *The Post-Soviet Wars: Rebellion, Ethnic Conflict and Nationhood in the Caucasus*. New York: NYU Press.

CHAPTER 2

# History and Ecology of Malaria in the Caucasus

**Abstract** This chapter explores the history of malaria in the Caucasus. Devastating epidemics of *Plasmodium vivax* (*P. vivax*) were quite common during the early decades of the twentieth century. Aggressive Soviet public health measures helped control outbreaks but the disease persisted until the pesticide DDT became available in the 1950s. As the Soviet Union entered its later years the expansion of the informal economy facilitated a return to a more traditional ethnic and kinship-based social order in the Caucasus. These developments were particularly noticeable in Karabakh due to its unique geography as an Armenian enclave inside the political territory of Azerbaijan.

By the late 1980s, ethnic separatism combined with communal violence to generate outflows of refugees and prolonged interruptions in public health prevention and vector control programs.

**Keywords** Malaria • Caucasus • Public Health History

## 2.1 The Caucasus

The Caucasus region consists of a mountainous land bridge that links Europe and Asia, occupied by dozens of distinct ethnic groups. The combination of rugged geography, strategic geopolitical importance and ethnic complexity has given the region a good deal of historical mystique, as


K. Hirschfeld et al., *New Wars and Old Plagues*,
https://doi.org/10.1007/978-3-031-31143-7_2

well as longstanding patterns of violence and instability (Broers 2021; Croissant 1998; de Waal 2013; King 2008; Tishkov 1997; Zurcher 2007). Since the nineteenth century, various imperial powers—including Great Britain, Russia, Turkey and Iran—have tried to control the region and forcibly assimilate its diverse ethnic groups into their expanding empires, but with little success. Russia's failed territorial incursions into the Caucasus in the late 1800s led to chronic violence, with "wholesale destruction of villages," and widespread torture of resistant populations (King 2008: 76). Russian troops also engaged in repeated bouts of ethnic and religious cleansing, and a number of Muslim villages were forcibly depopulated in the 1860s (King 2008: 94).

In the late nineteenth century, the ethnic composition of the Karabakh region was predominantly Armenian while the surrounding territories were composed of ethnic Tatar (Turkic) populations (Saparov 2012; Russian Empire Census n.d.). The census results from 1886 and 1897 indicate that the composition of the territories and major cities was fluid during this time (Russian Empire Census n.d.; NK Census 2005). This fluidity is reflected in the instability of the region due to tensions and fighting between the Russian and Ottoman Empires and the shifting relationships between the Ottoman Turks and Armenian residents in the Eastern Ottoman Empire (Saparov 2012). After the end of World War I and the collapse of the Russian and Ottoman Empires, a period of transition saw the brief formation of a Transcaucasian state, followed by the newly independent states of Armenia and Azerbaijan. The international borders of these states followed the Russian and Ottoman boundaries, and the territory of Karabakh became an issue of immediate debate among surrounding states. Episodes of violence and destruction occurred, shifting the population demographics in the region (Saparov 2012; de Waal 2013).

Beginning in the 1920s, Soviet officials sought to divide the Caucasus into ethnofederal units ranked hierarchically into three administrative categories. As Broers has described, "Each tier possessed corresponding attributes of statehood in descending order, with union republics possessing a formal right of self determination" (2021: 24). These tiers included SSRs (Soviet Socialist Republics), ASSRs (Autonomous Soviet Socialist Republics) and AO (Administrative Oblasts) (Zurcher 2007: 25).

Armenia and Azerbaijan were both SSRs, and were considered semi-sovereign states, at least in theory. Each SSR had its own government, military and constitution. ASSRs were administrative sub-units located within the boundaries of SSRs but populated by ethnic minorities. Chechnya, Dagestan and Ossetia were all ASSRs during the Soviet era. In 1923 Karabakh was formally declared one of two AO (Administrative Oblasts) located within the larger SSR of Azerbaijan, and became known as NKAO (Nagorno-Karabakh Administrative Oblast). The second semi-autonomous region located within the AZSSR (Azerbaijan Soviet Socialist Republic) was the southern territory of Nakhichevan, which was transferred by Turkey to the USSR as part of a treaty negotiated in the early 1920s (Broers 2021).

One goal of these administrative divisions was to reduce opposition to Soviet rule by dividing ethnic territories across ethnofederal units. As Broers stated with respect to the Armenian and Azerbaijani SSRs, "each republic's largest minority belonged to the other's nationality" (Broers 2021: 24). This gave the USSR a potential "fifth column" to activate against an unruly SSR government who might seek too much independence from the Soviet center. Michael Croissant has also described the formation of the NKAO as resulting in Stalin's "divide and rule" principle during his time as Soviet Commissar for Nationalities during the 1920s (Croissant 1998: 20).

## 2.2 Malaria in the Caucasus

Contemporary population health researchers may be surprised to learn that northern latitudes can be quite hospitable to malaria parasites. As historian Randy Packard has detailed, the designation of malaria as a tropical disease is a recent practice that came about following the successful eradication of temperate or seasonal *P. vivax* from northern regions in Europe in the mid-twentieth century (2007). The most severe form of malaria—*P. falciparum*—is a true tropical disease and cannot overwinter in northern climates. *P. vivax*, however, is an ancestral temperate strain that developed a remarkable ability to hibernate in the human body during winter months (White 2011). It re-emerges in the spring when mosquitos begin to hatch. In northern Russia, specialized arctic strains of *P. vivax* have been known to incubate in the human body for over a year (Johnson 1988).

Seasonal *P. vivax* malaria is much less likely to be fatal than tropical *P. falciparum*, but the disease can create significant morbidity, especially in agricultural populations during planting and harvest seasons (Bassat et al. 2016; Snowden 2006). In the memorable words of Sonia Shah,

> [V]ivax malaria … was not a killer. Rather it enslaved its victims, imposing a constant and unrelenting tax in blood. The convulsions of fever and chills arrived every summer and fall, as soon as the first mosquitoes fed on the blood of an obliviously relapsing carrier of dormant parasites. *P. vivax* infected the placentas of growing fetuses. Infected babies withered, with stunted immune defenses that rendered them vulnerable to diarrhea and pneumonia. Under the spell of chronic vivax infection, grown men and women weakened to the point that their ambitions drained away and they became anemically prone and wan, just vital enough to make more blood cells available for a later parasite feed. (Shah 2010: 32)

For these reasons, societies with uncontrolled *P. vivax* often have high rates of food shortages, poverty and economic stress (Sachs and Malaney 2002; Litsios 2002; Shah 2010; Snowden 2006). Because of its unique qualities as a blood parasite, malaria infection negatively impacts overall immunity, especially for young children (Anvikar et al. 2020; Bassat et al. 2016). High rates of *P. vivax* infection also increase overall mortality from all infectious diseases. In his analysis of malaria and demographic change in Italy, Frank Snowden stated, "Longevity and life expectancy data … revealed a terrible toll in radically foreshortened lives" (Snowden 2006: 15). Widespread malaria dramatically amplifies the health and mortality impact of many childhood diseases. One study in Malaysia, for instance, revealed that "disrupting malaria transmission sent other infectious diseases—diarrhea, dysentery, nephritis, accesses, tuberculosis, convulsions—plummeting as well" (Shah 2010: 178). A promising vaccine has been developed for *P. falciparum* malaria, but there is still no vaccine for *P. vivax* Drug treatments can be complicated due to ancestral genetic adaptations like G6PD deficiency (Carter and Mendis 2002). *P. vivax* is under-researched compared with *P. falciparum*, even though it is the most common form of malaria with an estimated 2.5 billion people considered at risk worldwide (Bassat et al. 2016).

## 2.3 Early Public Health Work in the Caucasus

One of the most significant obstacles limiting Russia's imperial incursions into the Caucasus in the 1800s was the presence of widespread epidemic malaria (Hackett 1937; King 2008). Malaria was very common throughout Europe and the Caucasus in the nineteenth and early twentieth centuries (see Fig. 2.1 for a historic map of malaria case density in the Caucasus).

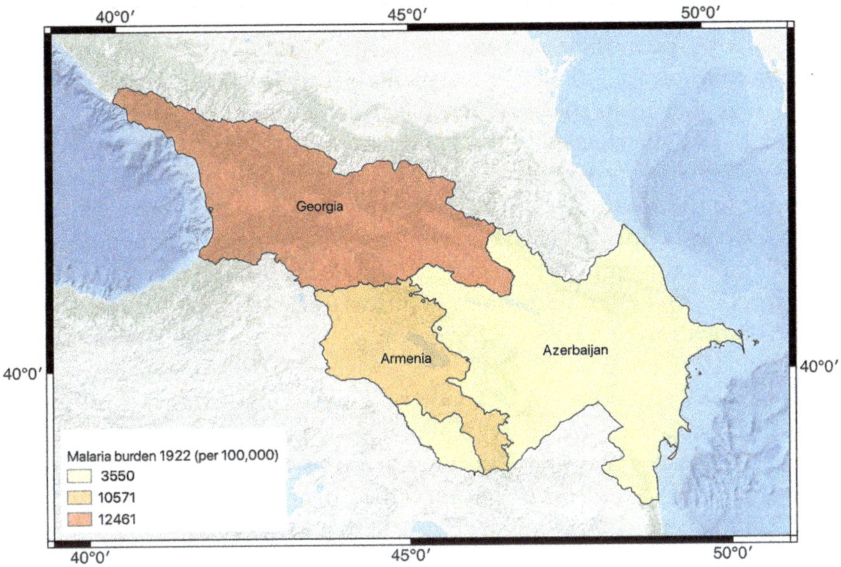


**Fig. 2.1** Map of malaria case density in the Caucasus 1920s. (Data is taken from League of Nations Malaria Commission reports, 1920s)

Malariologist L.W. Hackett once described the disease as "a great lake inundating all of Europe" (Hackett 1937: 3). Seasonal epidemics were especially devastating in the lowland Kura and Araks River valleys in the early decades of the twentieth century. In 1913 an unnamed public health officer described a "malignant" form of malaria widespread along the Volga River, with over five million cases per year estimated to occur in the region. The author asserted that no province in Russia was free of the disease, but cases appeared to be most heavily concentrated in the south-eastern part of the country. "The slow flow of the Russian rivers," the officer wrote, "creates numerous swamps along the borders of the rivers, and this circumstance, if accompanied by excessive heat during the summer months, is the cause of the presence of millions of mosquitoes" (Public Health Reports 1913: 207). In his report, he concluded that malaria was the "chief obstacle to successful colonization of the Caucasus and Turkestan" and overall "the cause of serious injury to the economic welfare of the population" due to its seasonal impact on agricultural labor (Public Health Reports 1913: 207).

In the early 1920s another report estimated malaria was a "widely prevalent … scourge in the Caucasus republics … and … the most important of all communicable diseases in Armenia" (Public Health Reports 1924: 223). A report from the League of Nations Malaria Commission noted that in 1923 malaria cases in the USSR were estimated to be over 13 million, whereas before World War I they averaged only around 3.5 million per year. In the southern Caucasus over one million people were estimated to be seasonally infected "most of whom were not receiving medical treatment" due to the high cost of quinine (Public Health Reports 1924: 224). In districts with high rates of malaria, it was not uncommon for up to 40% of the population to be affected in spring planting and fall harvest seasons (Johnson 1988: 34).

The USSR experienced a series of devastating famines during the 1920s, accompanied by epidemics of typhoid, typhus and cholera that spread into Eastern Europe (League of Nations 1922; Tarassévitch 1922). In 1925 the *British Medical Journal* linked the rapid increase in epidemic malaria in Russia to "vast movements of the population due to famine" as well as "climate conditions favoring the mosquito" (British Medical Journal 1925). In other words, the combination of increased population movements and increased population vulnerability led to explosive epidemics. Russia's post war outbreak soon spread internationally with cases exported to England, Germany and even far northern arctic regions (Hackett 1937: 2).

This pattern is common with *P. vivax*, which can have major fluctuations in virulence and prevalence configured by environmental conditions, varying population immunity and underlying population health (Hackett 1937). The disease usually produces mild symptoms in familiar populations, but can be deadly to new arrivals, undernourished hosts or vulnerable migrants. This is one of the reasons malaria created barriers to foreign colonization in the Caucasus: invading forces inevitably included soldiers with no prior exposure and these individuals suffered debilitating malaria infections while local populations were still able to fight. Fluctuations in weather patterns also interrupted seasonality of *P. vivax*, so that collective immunity was never fully established in the Caucasus, and devastating epidemics could appear after years of minor outbreaks (Johnson 1988; Hackett 1937).

## 2.4 The Caucasus: Ethnicity and Health in the Soviet Era

The Soviet Union completed its takeover of the Caucasus region in 1924, and immediately began campaigns to control infectious diseases and to subjugate the unruly ethnic groups that had historically proven so resistant to colonization. At this time, the population of NGK was predominantly Armenian. The first Soviet period census of the region was in 1926. The NGK region was composed of 125,300 residents. Of these, 89% were ethnic Armenian, 10% Turkic and the remaining were Russians. Several

surrounding villages and cities (including Shusha) were composed of ethnic Azerbaijan residents (NK Census 2005). As Broers has pointed out, the original borders of the Nagorny-Karabakh Administrative Oblast (NKAO) were designed to maximize separation of ethnic Armenians and Azeris (2021). The 1926 census, for instance, revealed the population of NKAO to be almost 90% Armenian in an area that represented approximately 5% of the Soviet Republic of Azerbaijan (AZSSR) (2021: 26).

In the 1930s, ethnic groups in the region were targeted for aggressive cultural "modernization" by Soviet authorities, and these programs included forced suppression of many ancestral cultural practices. Traditional subsistence practices, marriage patterns, clan affiliations, and religious practice were denounced by Soviet authorities as "crimes of custom" punishable by property confiscation, fines or prison (King 2008: 190). Ongoing resistance to Soviet control eventually led to wholesale deportation of thousands of Chechens, Balkars, Ingush and other groups from their ancestral lands to barren regions of Central Asia (King 2008; Tishkov 2004: 23). More than 300,000 Chechens and 80,000 Ingush were forcibly relocated in the 1940s, and their depopulated villages were resettled by Russian migrants, increasing local pressures for assimilation and Russification (King 2008).

Ethnic populations remaining in the Caucasus were eventually assimilated into quasi-ethnic administrative states that tolerated minor expressions of identity but outlawed any real challenges to secular Soviet homogenization. As Christopher Zurcher described, "On the surface, the Soviet type sovereign nation-states that were created as building blocks of the Soviet Union looked 'modern' but as with many other Soviet modernization projects, they were, in fact, more of a simulacrum of modernity" (2007: 31).

Soviet public health programs were developed with similar ideology of authoritarian modernization. Health campaigns in the first and second Five Year Plans were designed to rapidly assimilate rural areas under Soviet rule. Much emphasis was placed on the construction of hospitals and health facilities, and the creation of favorable reports detailing rapid progress in the control of preventable infectious diseases (Cockerham 1999). In some instances these Soviet public health efforts were "simulacra" or artificial monuments that reflected the ideology of health modernization but were ultimately bereft of key resources (Feshbach and Friendly 1992; Garrett 2000).

Malaria was not subject to the same level of politicization as Soviet campaigns against typhus, plague or cholera (Cockerham 1999; Johnson 1988). Instead, Soviet malariologists undertook complex environmental engineering and drainage projects designed to reduce seasonal flooding along the Volga basin and limit breeding grounds for anopheles mosquitos. There were also elaborate engineering projects in Armenia near the border with Turkey designed to funnel surface water into large waterways, eventually draining into the Araks River.[1] These efforts improved the agricultural production and reduced the pools and waterways used by the anopheles mosquito vectors. These efforts were paired with programs to improve housing, screen windows and limit outdoor sleeping (a common practice in peasant communities in summer months). Medical stations were established to provide regular doses of quinine to rural peasants in order to eliminate dormant parasites hidden in human bodies, but with mixed success (Tchnesova 1998).

The key innovation that finally led to lasting malaria control and eradication was the development of DDT, an insecticide that became available shortly after World War II (Shah 2010). At this time, political leaders in the United States and Europe recognized the devastating impact of malaria on military operations during the war. The German army, for instance, intentionally engineered an epidemic of malaria in Italy by flooding marshlands with brackish water to create expansive breeding grounds for the mosquito *A. labranchiae*. They also confiscated Italy's stockpiles of antimalaria drugs before retreating from the region at the end of the war. The resulting epidemic infected over 100,000 people (Shah 2010: 215). Malaria also impacted US military operations in the Pacific and decimated troops in New Guinea and Guadalcanal "felling more soldiers than enemy combat" (Shah 2010: 215).

DDT was far more effective than previous generations of chemical pesticides because of its environmental persistence. It was cheap to manufacture and did not require an extensive workforce since spraying could be done only once per season due to its remarkable persistence in the environment. As malariologist Paul Russell stated in 1952, "The special virtue of these insecticides [like DDT] is their lasting effectiveness. Because they remain lethal to mosquitoes many months after they are applied, they make it possible to wrest a region from the insects and hold it against reinvasion" (1952: 23).

Widespread use of DDT led to a decline in malaria cases in Italy from over 400,000 per year in 1950 to fewer than 1000 in 1951 (Russell 1952). Similar declines occurred all over the Pacific, Latin America and in the United States. India's caseload declined from seventy-five million before World War II to fewer than 100,000 in the mid-1950s (Shah 2010: 229). In Venezuela all homes in malarious regions were sprayed and the disease was "suppressed to insignificance" in just a few years (Russell 1952: 24). The Soviet Union also participated in these global efforts and finally achieved malaria eradication in the Caucasus in the early 1960s (Tchnesova 1998).

DDT was outlawed in the 1970s, and after that time malaria control in the USSR was maintained through regular disease surveillance and inspection of waterways.

Human mobility was limited during this time and Soviet borders were generally closed, so the potential for reintroduction of malaria to the Caucasus was low. These prevention and control measures were sufficient to maintain the region's malaria-free status until the conflict period of the early 1990s.

## 2.5 Late Soviet Political Economy: Setting the Stage for Conflict

By the 1970s the centralized economic system of the USSR began to take on very different qualities than those envisioned by the original architects of the Soviet system. Specifically, the formal economic sector became increasingly hollowed out and the majority of goods and services were siphoned into exchange networks organized by entrepreneurs in the informal economy (Garrett 2000; King 2008; Ledneva 1998; Zurcher 2007). This happened for a variety of reasons, but most significantly from the inability of the centralized economic system to supply industries or individuals with basic goods essential for survival. In the Soviet system, factory managers were faced with rigid production quotas, even though the state could not provide the raw materials required for manufacturing. Criticizing supply chain failures was risky—equivalent to expressing political dissent—so a variety of improvised solutions developed that maintained the facade of Soviet socialist success, but further eroded any vestiges of institutional honesty or compliance with the dictates of the central government.

These improvised solutions included elaborate systems of informal exchange organized by extended kin groups and hierarchical patronage networks. As Friedrich and Brzezinski described, "[Soviet] Managers ... maximize their achievements by taking shortcuts on standards or by actually falsifying records; they organize informal arrangements among themselves, based practically on bribery, to avoid control and to exchange necessary items... " (1965: 212). Over time, these practices expanded into proxy expressions of political dissent. One anthropologist stated succinctly, "the [Soviet] regimes were constantly undermined by internal resistance and hidden forms of sabotage at all system levels" (Verdery 1996: 20). Daniel Chirot described how Soviet economies turn into "vast patronage pyramids" due to the fact that "each [factory] leader and administrator in the chain of command was trying to build up a personal clique of followers who could be counted on for support..." (1994: 162).

A number of scholars have described the effect of these developments on Soviet institutions and Soviet ideology in the 1970s and 1980s (Berger 1986; Chirot 1994; Davis 1989; Feshbach and Friendly 1992; Gleason 1997; Koehler and Zurcher 2003a; Kolakowski 1992; Malia 1994; Verdery 1996). A common theme in these analyses is the inevitable loss of faith that resulted from widening gaps between official versions of Soviet reality (as represented in state-controlled mass media) and observable dynamics of everyday life. Leszek Kołakowski described this duality as highlighting "the ridiculous emptiness of the official ideology," and accelerating popular disaffection with Soviet rule (Kolakowski 1992: 46).

The ideological decline of the late Soviet period further energized the informal economy as a space of political resistance and entrepreneurial success. Political dissent remained criminalized, but diversion of goods from the state sector to private hands became a popular and lucrative activity—a profitable way to undermine the repressive apparatus of the state. Many analyses of this time period describe a powerful "shadow economy" operating within various sectors of the Soviet system that served to redirect valuable goods (including military equipment and construction materials) into private hands (Chirot 1994; Dudwick 1997; Gall and De Waal 1997; de Waal 2013; Handelman 1995; King 2008; Koehler and Zurcher 2003a; Koehler and Zurcher 2003b; Ledneva 1998; Zurcher 2007).

In the Caucasus region, local Party leaders were described by one journalist as "feudal lords who paid homage to the court in Moscow but ran their own fiefdoms at home" (de Waal 2013: 146). In Armenia, trusted kinship and family connections became an essential tool for accessing scarce resources (Dudwick 1997). Historian Charles King described how Soviet policies—specifically the inefficiencies of centralized planning and the development of a parallel informal economy—unintentionally revitalized the traditional clan-based social organization of the Caucasus,

> These features of Soviet life strengthened familial and patron-client relationships, and the networks of debt and responsibility that are often given the label 'clans.' Clan networks were traditionally an important element of Caucasus society, both north and south of the mountains … One would have expected the importance of such premodern social conventions to decline with time, but in many ways the Soviet system strengthened them. In an economy of scarcity social networks were critical in providing access to goods and power, and the clan networks of the past served that purpose. (King 2008: 202)

Transactions in the informal economy take place within the territorial boundaries of an established nation-state, but they occur outside of political space, with no government oversight or control (Parrott 1997). This creates challenges in that there is no one in authority to enforce contracts or punish thieves—essential activities for maintaining trust and continuity in systems of exchange. Personal relationships, especially kin relations, become extremely important in this context. Kinship and family connections provide a pre-existing set of obligations that are life long and easily extended in ways that support collective business endeavors operating outside control of the state. As anthropologist Nora Dudwick described during her field research in Armenia, "The pervasive shortages [of the Soviet economy] encouraged a sense of competition and mutual distrust, further increasing the importance of the family as a dependable and trustworthy safety net" (1997: 74).

The importance of these kin-based patronage networks became even more acute following a devastating earthquake in Armenia in the winter of 1988. This natural disaster leveled the cities of Spitak and Stepanavan, and an estimated 1500 villages and 35,000 private dwellings were destroyed (de Waal 2013: 65). Hundreds of thousands of people were left homeless and approximately 25,000 died. Reports of widespread corruption—including diversion of essential humanitarian relief and reconstruction supplies by Soviet officials—led to further intensification of anti-Soviet sentiment throughout the region (de Waal 2013: 65; Dudwick 1997: 107).

As Soviet legitimacy declined in the 1980s, ethnicity and nationalism re-emerged to structure social and economic relations in the Caucasus. These trends increased ethnic tensions and separatist groups like the Karabakh Committee soon emerged as a "shadow government eclipsing formal Soviet institutions" (Broers 2021: 162). A visit by Soviet Premier Mikhail Gorbachev to Armenia a few days after the earthquake further inflamed tensions as he spoke out against Armenian nationalism and derided the leaders of the Karabakh Committee as "unscrupulous people, demagogues, adventurers, corrupt people, black shirts who were hungry for power" (de Waal 2013: 66). The separatist Karabakh Committee was arrested and sent to Moscow, further alienating local populations and fueling the expansion of the informal economy as a space of political resistance and cultural preservation.

Several assessments of the Karabakh conflict identify Soviet era extended kin networks, patronage systems and their respective activities in the "shadow economy" as key contributors to the violence that developed in the late 1980s (de Waal 2013; Dudwick 1997; Kaldor 2007; Koehler and Zurcher 2003a; Zurcher 2007). According to Thomas de Waal, the capital flowing through the informal economy in 1988 was estimated to be ten billion rubles in Azerbaijan and 14 billion in Armenia (de Waal 2013: 153). When Soviet institutions began to falter, underworld entrepreneurs took advantage of the power vacuum to expand their operations. Since much of the informal economy was organized on ethnic lines, this economic competition became manifest as ethnic conflict. As de Waal stated, "…what may have deepened the anxieties of the Karabakh Armenians in the 1970s and 1980s was that they were losing out to a more powerful Azerbaijani networks in the underground economy: as a minority they were not strong enough to claim a large slice of the pie" (de Waal 2013: 153).

Koehler and Zurcher have also used the term "ethnic entrepreneurs" to describe the fusion of political, economic and ethnic groups in the aftermath of the Soviet collapse (Koehler and Zurcher 2003b: 12). "State weakness," they argue, "... unblocks access to resources and power ... A key resource in power struggles can be ethnicity. Political entrepreneurs thus often turn into ethnic entrepreneurs—they appeal to real or perceived threats and injustices in order to mobilize support" (2003a: 12). The specific term used to describe these individuals is "biznesmen-patrioty" or "patriotic businessmen." These were individuals who maintained lucrative patronage systems within Soviet economies, organized through personal connections and extended kin groups (2003a: 149). They also used their patronage positions to finance and develop the fledging institutions of post-Soviet states.

Unfortunately, these processes contributed to the amplification of ethnic conflict during and after the Soviet collapse (Koehler and Zurcher 2003a). *Biznesmen* increasingly used their influence and resources to support separatist movements and ethnonationalist militias (Koehler and Zurcher 2003:149; Zurcher 2007). In the Karabakh region, the exact nature of the *biznes* operated by patriotic businessmen is unclear. But the region's status as a producer of desirable luxury goods (including valuable citrus fruit and brandy) during the Soviet period likely played a role. Thomas de Waal has also reported rumors of marijuana plantations operating in Karabakh (de Waal 2013: 153). In neighboring Georgia the 1980s were described as "a period of especially rapid growth in the shadow economy ... since produce from the Abkhazian agricultural sector, including tea, tobacco, wine and citrus fruits, brought huge profits on the Soviet market" (Zurcher 2007: 121).

The geography of the southern Caucasus—consisting of high mountain passes that form a critical land bridge between Europe and Asia—also makes the entire region valuable as smuggling territory. Transit corridors in mountainous regions are limited, and any group that controlled a remote mountain pass would be able to collect revenues for guaranteeing safe passage for valuable cargo. These practices had a long history in the Caucasus. As one historian noted, "Until the late nineteenth century the borders separating the many different political entities in the Caucasus were often opportunities for extraction—collecting tolls for safe passage ... The goal of any political power was to control the locus of extraction, such as a key bridge, port, mountain pass or fortress" (King 2008: 21).

## Note

1. During our field site visits to Armenia, several elderly residents remembered the improved effects of these water works.

## References


Anvikar, Anupkumar, Anna Maria, Asha van Eijk, Kamlesh J. Shah, Steven A. Upadhyay, Ankita J. Sullivan, Jaykumar M. Patel, Suchi Tyagi Joshi, Ranvir Singh, Jane M. Carlton, Himanshu Gupta, and Samuel C. Wassmer. 2020. Clinical and Epidemiological Characterization of Severe *Plasmodium vivax* Malaria in Gujarat, India. *Virulence* 11 (1): 730–738.

Bassat, Quique, Mar Velarde, Ivo Mueller, Jessica Lin, Toby Leslie, C. Chansuda Wongsrichanalai, and J. Kevin Baird. 2016. Key Knowledge Gaps for *Plasmodium vivax* Control and Elimination. *American Journal of Tropical Medicine and Hygiene* 95 (suppl 6): 62–71.

Berger, Peter. 1986. *The Capitalist Revolution: Fifty Propositions about Prosperity, Equality and Liberty*. New York: Basic Books.

British Medical Journal. 1925. The World Epidemiology of 1924. 2(3376): 483–484.

Broers, Laurence. 2021. *Armenia and Azerbaijan: Anatomy of a Rivalry*. Edinburgh: Edinburgh University Press.

Carter, Richard, and Kamini N. Mendis. 2002. Evolutionary and Historical Aspects of the Burden of Malaria. *Clinical Microbiology Reviews* 15 (4): 564–594.

Chirot, Daniel. 1994. *Modern Tyrants: The Power and Prevalence of Evil in Our Age*. New York: The Free Press.

Cockerham, William. 1999. *Health and Social Change in Russia and Eastern Europe*. New York: Routledge.

Croissant, Michael. 1998. *The Armenia-Azerbaijan Conflict: Causes and Implications*. Westport, CT: Praeger.

Davis, Christopher. 1989. The Soviet Health Care System: A National Health Service in a Socialist Society. In *Success and Crisis in National Health Systems: A Comparative Approach*, ed. Mark Field, 233–264. Routledge.

de Waal, Thomas. 2013. *Black Garden: Armenia and Azerbaijan Through Peace and War*. New York: New York University Press.

Dudwick, Nora. 1997. Political Transformation in Post-communist Armenia: Images and Realities. In *Conflict, Cleavage and Change in Central Asia and the Caucasus*, ed. Karen Dawisha and Bruce Parrott, 69–109. Cambridge: Cambridge University Press.

Feshbach, Murray, and Alfred Friendly. 1992. *Ecocide in the USSR: Health and Nature under Siege*. New York: Basic Books.

Friedrich, Carl, and Brzezinski, Zbigniew. 1965. [1956] *Totalitarian Dictatorship and Autocracy*. New York: Frederick Praeger.

Gall, Carlotta, and Thomas De Waal. 1997. *Chechnya: A Small Victorious War*. London: Pan Books.

Garrett, Laurie. 2000. *Betrayal of Trust: The Collapse of Global Public Health.* New York: Hyperion.

Gleason, Abbott. 1997. *Totalitarianism: The Inner History of the Cold War.* New York: Oxford University Press.

Hackett, Lewis W. 1937. *Malaria in Europe: An Ecological Survey.* London: Oxford University Press.

Handelman, Stephen. 1995. *Comrade Criminal: Russia's New Mafiya.* New Haven: Yale University Press.

Johnson, Richard. 1988. *Malaria and Malaria Control in the USSR, 1917–1941.* PhD thesis,. Georgetown University Department of History.

Kaldor, Mary. 2007. Oil and Conflict: The Case of Nagorno-Karabakh. In *Oil Wars*, ed. Mary Kaldor, Terry Lynn Karl, and Yahia Said, 157–182. London: Pluto Press.

King, Charles. 2008. *The Ghost of Freedom: A History of the Caucasus.* Oxford: Oxford University Press.

Koehler, Jan, and Christoph Zurcher. 2003a. Introduction. In *Potentials of Disorder: New Approaches to Conflict Analysis*, ed. Jan Koehler and Christoph Zurcher, 1–12. Manchester: Manchester University Press.

———. 2003b. The Art of Losing the State: Weak Empire to Weak Nation-State Around Nagorno-Karabakh. In *Potentials of Disorder: New Approaches to Conflict Analysis*, ed. Jan Koehler and Christoph Zurcher, 145–173. Manchester: Manchester University Press.

Kolakowski, Leszek. 1992. Amidst Moving Ruins. *Daedelus* 121: 43–56.

League of Nations. 1922. *Report on the Health Situation in Eastern Europe.* Retrieved from RG 90 Records of the United States Public Health Service. National Archives and Records Administration, College Park, Maryland July 2019.

Ledneva, Alena. 1998. *Russia's Economy of Favors: Blat, Networking and Informal Exchange.* Cambridge: Cambridge University Press.

Litsios, Socrates. 2002. Malaria Control and the Future of International Public Health. In *The Contextual Determinants of Malaria*, ed. Elizabeth Casman and Hadi Dowlatabadi, 292–328. Washington, DC: Resources for the Future.

Malia, Martin. 1994. *The Soviet Tragedy: A History of Socialism in Russia, 1917–1991.* New York: The Free Press.

Nagorno Karabakh (NK) Census. 2005. About the First Population Census of the Nagorno Karabakh Republic 2005. http://census.stat-nkr.am/nkr/pervaya_perepis.pdf. Accessed April 2021.

Packard, Randall. 2007. *The Making of a Tropical Disease.* Baltimore, Maryland: Johns Hopkins University Press.

Parrott, Bruce. 1997. Perspectives on Postcommunist Democratization. In *Conflict, Cleavage and Change in Central Asia and the Caucasus*, ed. Karen Dawisha and Bruce Parrott, 1–39. Cambridge: Cambridge University Press.

Public Health Reports. 1913. Malaria in Russia: Its Prevalence and Geographic Distribution. 28 (5): 206–207.

———. 1924. Prevalence of Disease: Foreign and Insular, 39(5): 220–230.
Russell, Paul. 1952. The Eradication of Malaria. *Scientific American* 186 (6): 22–25.
Russian Empire Census. n.d. Azerbaijan Soviet Socialist Republic. http://www.ethno-kavkaz.narod.ru/rnazerbaijan.html.
Sachs, Jeffrey, and Pia Malaney. 2002. The Economic and Social Burden of Malaria. *Nature*, 2002 Feb 7; 415 (6872): 680–685. https://doi.org/10.1038/415680a.
Saparov, Arséne. 2012. Why Autonomy? The Making of Nagorno-Karabakh Autonomous Region 1918–1925. *Europe-Asia Studies* 64 (2): 281–323.
Shah, Sonia. 2010. *The Fever: How Malaria Has Ruled Mankind for 500,000 Years*. New York: Farrar, Strauss and Giroux. Ibooks edition.
Snowden, Frank. 2006. *The Conquest of Malaria: Italy, 1900–1962*. New Haven, CT: Yale University Press.
Tarassévitch, Professor L. 1922. *Epidemics in Russia Since 1914*. Report to the Health Committee of the League of Nations. Retrieved from RG 90 Records of the United States Public Health Service, National Archives and Records Administration College Park, Maryland.
Tchnesova, L. 1998. Socio-economic and scientific premises for forming the strategies against malaria in Russia under Soviet power. *Parassitologia* 40: 103–108.
Tishkov, Valery. 1997. *Ethnicity, Nationalism and Conflict in and After the Soviet Union: The Mind Aflame*. London: Sage Publications.
White, M. 2011. Determinants of Relapse Periodicity in Plasmodium vivax Malaria. *Malaria Journal* https://malariajournal.biomedcentral.com/track/pdf/10.1186/1475-2875-10-297. Accessed 18 June 2020.
Zurcher, Christopher. 2007. *The Post-Soviet Wars: Rebellion, Ethnic Conflict and Nationhood in the Caucasus*. New York: NYU Press.

CHAPTER 3

# The Karabakh Conflict, 1988–1994

**Abstract** This chapter provides a chronological overview of the Karabakh conflict, beginning with the development of ethnic violence in the late 1980s and continuing through the collapse of the Soviet Union in the early 1990s. The initial phase of unrest in Karabakh was met with Soviet military aggression, particularly against Armenian villages that were known to support separatists. Thousands of Armenian and Azeri refugees fled Karabakh and relocated to urban areas where their stories of persecution stoked retaliatory violence. As Soviet power began to wane, military equipment from the Soviet army began to filter into different militia groups, fueling more intense violence that rapidly accelerated into nation-state warfare after the collapse of the USSR. As the war intensified a severe economic and humanitarian crisis unfolded that left thousands of refugees without heat, hot water or medical services throughout the region.

**Keywords** Karabakh • Conflict • Political collapse • Ethnic violence

## 3.1 Ethnicity and Nationalism

Population data from the Soviet era indicates that the Karabakh region was slowly urbanizing in the second half of the twentieth century, and the ethnic mix was shifting to a higher proportion of Azeri residents. Urban populations increased from 26,973 to 97,410 from 1959 to 1989, while


K. Hirschfeld et al., *New Wars and Old Plagues*,
https://doi.org/10.1007/978-3-031-31143-7_3

rural populations decreased from 103,433 to 90,353 during the same time (NGK Census 2005). Reports suggest that a push to move ethnic Azerbaijanis into NGK was initiated by the Azerbaijani SSR in the space left by the changing demographics in NGK. This is supported by the increase in Azerbaijani population from 14 to 22% from 1959 to 1989. During the same time, the ethnic Armenian population in NGK decreased from 84 to 77%. The opening of factories by Azerbaijan in areas in and around NGK is thought to have occurred to entice ethnic Azeris into these regions (Horizon 2019).

Throughout the Soviet era Armenians repeatedly petitioned Moscow for a new political geography of ethnic reunification. Lingering cultural trauma from the early twentieth-century genocide added urgency to these requests.[1] When Soviet power began to falter in the late 1980s, Armenian nationalists again pressed Soviet leaders to reassign Karabakh to the territory of Armenia. When these efforts were unsuccessful, tensions increased. Residents of NGK formally passed a resolution to reunify with the Armenian SSR in the summer of 1988 (de Waal 2013). They subsequently held a national referendum on independence and soon formed the Republic of Artsakh.

The contraction of Soviet power in the late 1980s, however, meant that the Soviet response to Armenian separatism was disorganized, heavy-handed and ill conceived (Croissant 1998; de Waal 2013). The expansive informal economy in the region also meant that local *biznesmen* were powerful enough to subvert Soviet power through informal channels and had sufficient resources and procurement networks to supply local militias with contraband weapons (Kaldor 2007; Kohler and Zurcher 2003b: 161). The waning of Soviet power also meant that longstanding patronage networks became destabilized, and valuable resources circulating in the informal economy could be considered up for grabs. As Nora Dudwick described,

> Despite the apparent bankruptcy of the state budget, there are enormous sums to be made during this period of rapid unpredictable change. Well-placed people are scrambling to secure their access to this wealth by buying and selling of state holdings which are being privatized, asserting control over natural resources, and establishing trade and production monopolies ... new authorities can demand which impunity whatever bribes or payments the market will bear. (1997: 90)

The violence that erupted in Karabakh was originally articulated in ethnic terms, but several scholars have argued that economic competition between rival entrepreneurs in the informal economy—*biznesmen-patrioty*—also played an important role (de Waal 2013; Koehler and Zurcher 2003; Zurcher 2007). As Koelher and Zurcher described, "…[T]he initial conflicts [in Karabakh] were not new nor about ethnic belonging. Instead, they were more about the control of lucrative segments of the 'shadow' economy by competing networks" (2003b: 149). Zurcher has also explored the links between Karabakh's early ethnic armies and pre-existing criminal groups operating in the informal economy. "They brought in an expertise in organizing violence … and quite often also a taste for fighting in the name of the nation" (2007: 216). He described similar patterns in the organization of violence in the neighboring Chechen and Georgian conflicts (2007: 216). The pattern of ethnic movements intensifying to form an "emergent substate" during periods of political collapse has been documented for a number of other regions experiencing separatist conflict in the 1990s (Mandic 2021).

According to one analysis, the ethnic dimension of the Karabakh conflict also emerged as a secondary effect of local marriage patterns (Dudwick 1997; Koehler and Zurcher 2003). Despite living in neighboring towns for decades of Soviet rule, an ethnic boundary was maintained between Armenians and Azeris through the preservation of ethnic intermarriage. These cultural practices were of minor importance during the secular Soviet period. But kin relations and religious practices became revitalized as Soviet power waned, and ethnic identity emerged as a key institution linking families together in networks of shared beliefs, traditions and trust. While there were examples of neighboring Azeri and Armenian families providing shelter and aid to one another during early outbreaks of ethnic violence, the geographic segregation created by ethnic removals and forced migration made such relationships increasingly difficult to sustain after 1991 (Goltz 1998).

## 3.2 Early Phase Conflict, 1988–1990

In the early phase of the conflict between 1988 and 1990, the territory of Karabakh was repeatedly assaulted by informal ethnic armies operating outside the Soviet system. This phase was low intensity, with poorly equipped militias engaging with other poorly equipped militias. Thomas Goltz described several of the early Azeri armed groups, for instance, as "composed more of extended families than soldiers" (1998: 150). Reports of ethnic violence in Karabakh, however, reverberated in the capital cities of Baku and Yerevan, leading to urban protests, riots and retaliatory pogroms. *Biznesmen-patrioty* increased their support for ethnic violence, mobilizing resources from diaspora communities and the "shadowy Azeri mafia" (Zurcher 2007). Broers has described this phase of intensifying ethnic violence as "a crucible forging a national identity in the capital [of Baku] where an alternative cosmopolitan identity was strongest" (Broers 2021: 133).

An ill-fated Soviet crackdown began in January 1990 with troops marching into Baku and killing over one hundred protestors. Communal violence was high and Armenian enclaves in Baku were targeted by angry mobs, leading to a mass exodus of refugees. The Armenian population of Baku declined from approximately 180,000 residents in 1989 to only 13,000 after the violence of "Black January" in 1990 (Broers 2021; de Waal 2013: 93).

The rapid exit of Armenians and Azeris from formerly cosmopolitan cities of Baku and Yerevan left each city ethnically homogenous and struggling to accommodate thousands of impoverished refugees. Karabakh remained multi-ethnic, but with internal segregation by town. Raiding, arson and hostage-taking between Armenian and Azeri villages soon became common (Broers 2021: 141). Refugees from Karabakh arrived in urban areas that were poorly equipped to provide them with housing, jobs or humanitarian assistance. As social services buckled under the strain of new arrivals, refugees became "a radicalizing force that fueled bloody inter communal clashes through 1990" (Croissant 1998: 28).

A group of Soviet officials also traveled to the Armenian enclave of Stepanakert where they were besieged by separatists. Annoyed by the display of ethnonational independence, the Soviets arrested a group of Armenian nationalists and also replaced the leadership of the Azeri Communist Party (de Waal 2013; Zurcher 2007). These actions intensified the growing convergence of anti-Soviet sentiment and ethnonational violence. Soviet soldiers also anticipated the impending fragmentation of the USSR and began informally selling high grade military weapons and supplies to various combatants in the Caucasus (Zurcher 2007: 217). Ethnic militias also attacked Soviet military installations in order to acquire rocket launchers, grenades and automatic rifles (de Waal 2013).

Between 1990 and 1991 the entire southern Caucasus region witnessed repeated rounds of low intensity conflict and heavy handed Soviet retaliation. At one point a joint operation between Azeri and Soviet forces called "Operation Ring" was launched to disarm Armenian militias and cut off support from rural enclaves. Armenian villages in Karabakh were encircled by Soviet and Azeri troops and residents were forcibly deported. Azeri settlers were then brought in to populate newly vacated houses and farmland.

At least 17 Armenian villages in the Karabakh region were targeted for forced depopulation during this time, with over 5000 Armenians deported and several dozen killed by Soviet and Azeri forces (de Waal 2013: 118). There were reports of Armenians trapped in villages without sufficient food, water or electricity for months at a time (de Waal 2013: 119). A few months later, Armenian forces succeeded in retaking some of these depopulated villages, forcing the recently settled Azeri residents to flee. Over time, these dynamics created "empty spaces, bereft of inhabitants" (Broers 2021: 141).

Repeated rounds of rural depopulation, exodus and resettlement also intensified the housing and humanitarian crisis in Armenia, which was still reeling from the effects of the 1988 earthquake. A 1991 USAID report noted over 400,000 Armenian earthquake victims were still "living in tents, garages and other makeshift shelters," and aid promised by the Soviet Union had failed to materialize (Vartain 1991). The "tragic situation" was further compounded by an influx of over 300,000 Armenian refugees fleeing violence in Azerbaijan and Karabakh. The report estimated Armenia was struggling with a population of 750,000 homeless people out of a total population of only 3.5 million. USAID officials working in Armenia summarized the complexities of providing humanitarian assistance in the late Soviet period as follows,

> The way the Soviet transportation and supply system was set up under Stalin (which is still operative today), all goods except air cargo coming into Armenia must go through the republics of either Azerbaijan or Georgia. All railroads (which carry most of Soviet goods) into Armenia go through those two republics. All commerce with the rest of the world must pass through the Soviet Union, Turkey or Iran. At present, Turkey and Iran are not viable routes, although a highway route through Turkey to the Black Sea is presently under negotiation. Highway transportation infrastructure in the former Soviet Union is not as well developed as in the West, and is much more subject to hijacking and other abuses than rail transport. … the Republic of Azerbaijan, through which most supplies have come during the last 70

> years, simply refuses to allow goods to pass into Armenia. Natural gas and other fuels from the Azeri oil fields are thus in very short supply, and other goods are diverted into both the Azeri economy and the hands of private, illegal groups and individuals … The Azerbaijani government remains in the hands of hard line 'former' communists, hostile to both Armenia and democracy, who are taking full advantage of their position in the supply chain to damage Armenia. The border between the two republics is in a state of civil war which the Center has done little to curtail. This complex combination of factors has produced shortages of everything except rocks and Armenians, both of which are plentiful in Armenia. (Vartain 1991)

## 3.3 Soviet Collapse and Nation-State Warfare, 1991–1994

Just a few months later the Soviet Union underwent its final collapse following a failed coup attempt against Premier Gorbachev. Almost immediately Armenia, Azerbaijan and Karabakh declared themselves independent nations. The semi-autonomous Azeri region of Nakhichevan elected former Soviet Central Committee member Heydar Aliyev as its Chairman, and according to one analyst he ruled the area "as his own private fiefdom, cultivating commercial ties with Turkey and Iran" (Croissant 1998: 90). Armenia acted quickly to retake several of the villages lost during Operation Ring.

The fragile new governments of Armenia and Azerbaijan also began enacting punishing sanctions against one another. Azerbaijan imposed an energy embargo that cut off Armenia's supplies of natural gas at the beginning of a freezing winter season. Within two weeks, life in Yerevan was "at a virtual standstill" (Croissant 1998: 45). Armenia's only nuclear power plant was still offline due to the earthquake and almost no imported goods were available due to the transportation blockade. To retaliate against Azerbaijan's energy embargo, Armenia cut off all access to the Azeri town of Xodjali, leaving the Azeri inhabitants with no electricity, heating oil or running water (Croissant 1998; Goltz 1998: 120).[2]

Around this time, USAID officials in Armenia began to complain about widespread theft and hijacking of supplies shipped through Russia and Georgia. Living conditions in the capital city continued to deteriorate. Power outages were common and heating fuel was scarce. One US medical professional working in Yerevan described conditions in January 1992 as follows,

> Presently we get three hours of electricity alternating with three hours off. The warmest my room/office gets is 60-65F and during the shut off period it gets down to 48-50F ... The general economic situation here is getting worse and worse. As a result of the price increases, the cost of living has increased at the very least by 10 fold while salaries have only been increased by 50%. Consumer goods and food stuffs are becoming increasingly incredibly priced. People are justly worried as to how they will make ends meet next month ... Unfortunately there is still room for the situation to get worse before it starts to get better ... (Fax sent from Stella Grigorian to Aryeh Cooperstock, Henryka Manes, Gabrielle Brook January 29 1992)

By the spring of 1992, Armenia managed to gain the upper hand in the conflict. Most Azeri civilians had been expelled from Karabakh, and Armenia seized enough territory to create a land bridge uniting the country into a single geographic unit. Some of this success was due to the fact that many Armenian military leaders had previously occupied high ranking posts in the Soviet army and were skilled professional soldiers. Soviet discrimination against Muslim republics like Azerbaijan meant Azeris who served in the Soviet army were rarely promoted to high rank and were instead relegated to the "notoriously undisciplined construction battalions" (Koehler and Zurcher 2003: 162). These dynamics led to disarray in the Azeri forces as professional solders did not want to serve "under the dubious command ... of warlords with no military education whatsoever" (Koehler and Zurcher 2003: 162). In spring 1992 the Azeri defense minister gave a speech to Parliament in which he described the conditions facing the country,

> We have no army at present. We called for 20,000 volunteers, but in real terms we have less than 5,000. The borders are weak, and even towns under attack have not bothered to fortify positions. There is no plan, no sense of tactics, no idea of what equipment is available or even who knows how to use it. (Quoted in Goltz 1998: 143–144)

Azerbaijan's internal conflicts and factionalism were exacerbated by the discovery of billions of dollars' worth of oil and gas reserves in the Caspian Sea. This drew the attention of multi-national oil companies who sent envoys to negotiate deals with Azeri leaders for exploration and pipeline construction (Goltz 1998).[3] Political office in Azerbaijan suddenly became more desirable and different factions began competing for the spoils of oil and gas concessions (Broers 2021). Russia remained involved in the conflict, allegedly playing both sides in order to maximize its own position and reassert its "traditional spheres of power" (de Waal 2013; Goltz 1998). Not long after taking office, Azerbaijan's President Elchibey accused Russia of "pitting different groups of our population against each other in order to prevent us from creating a truly independent state" (quoted in Goltz 1998: 146).

In spring 1992 there were reports of Armenian troops approaching Nakhichevan and the border area near Turkey. Russia immediately warned that if Turkey attempted to enter the conflict or demonstrated hostilities against Armenia it "could trigger a Third World War." Turkey was a NATO member and Russia still considered Armenia to be its regional and strategic ally (Croissant 1998: 82). There were also rumors that Iran was supporting a new Islamic party in Azerbaijan (Goltz 1998: 183).

In November 1992 a helicopter carrying Russian and Kazakh officials on their way to implement a peace deal was shot down in southern Karabakh, allegedly by Armenian fighters. Soon after, Azerbaijan's National Council voted to revoke Karabakh's status as an autonomous region and declare it a formal province of Azerbaijan (de Waal 2013: 176). Armenia retaliated by holding a referendum for Karabakh's independence and launching a major military offensive to regain lost territory (Croissant 1998). Soon after, Azeri saboteurs began attacking a key gas pipeline in Marneuili, a region of neighboring Georgia populated by Azeris. These energy disruptions left Armenia "in complete darkness" and without heat, phone service, cooking fuel or public transport during the coldest months of winter (Isaryan 1994). During the siege of Stepanakert, residents lived in basements with only candles for light, and urban residents had to hand carry water from distant springs (de Waal 2013: 188). In February 1993 USAID advisors issued a press release stating, "The humanitarian situation in Armenia is reaching critical proportions, as extreme shortages of fuel, food and medical supplies continue to define the daily lives of the Armenian people" (Marshall 1993).

Despite the energy crisis and destruction of key infrastructure, Armenia was able to retake a good deal of territory after Azeri warlord Surat Husseinov removed his troops from the strategic Kelbajar region in March 1993. Demoralized Azeri soldiers abandoned the town and hundreds of refugees were forced to travel along a snowy mountain road where many died of hypothermia (de Waal 2013: 224). In April the Armenian military opened a second offensive south of the Karabakh region and managed to seize control of 18 additional villages, some of which were located close to the Iranian border. Tens of thousands of Azeris fled the region and crossed the border into Turkey. The growing proximity of the conflict to geopolitical risk zones in Turkey and Iran led to increased pressure from the UN Security Council for a full cessation of hostilities (Croissant 1998: 87).

In May 1993 Surat Huseinov began attacking Azeri government forces when he attempted to seize weapons, ammunition and equipment from departing Russian soldiers in the city of Ganja. Huseinov told his troops to take control of all nearby villages, essentially holding them hostage to compel negotiations with President Elchibey. Elchibey responded by sending military helicopters to attack Huseinov's forces but without warning all three pilots suddenly switched sides, potentially paving the way for Huseinov to seize power with help from the armed forces (Goltz 1998). Huseinov's army then began marching toward Baku, threatening civil war. President Elchibey mysteriously disappeared around this time, leading some to speculate he was "drunk or drugged" while his government teetered on the brink of collapse (Goltz 1998: 364). A second Azeri military commander also staged a small rebellion in the Lenkoran region and declared a short lived autonomous "Talysh-Mugham Republic" (de Waal 2013: 227).

Azerbaijan's internal political fragmentation was eventually stabilized when former Soviet Central Committee member Heydar Aliyev maneuvered himself back into power following Elchibey's resignation in June 1993. One of Aliyev's first executive acts was to appoint warlord Surat Husseinov as Prime Minister, then cancel all of the oil contracts negotiated by President Elchibey (de Waal 2013). One former Azeri official complained to the *Los Angeles Times* that "feuding warlords have ousted two presidents and frustrated seven defense ministers in less than two years of independence" (*Los Angeles Times*, July 20, 1993).

The Armenian military took advantage of the internal fractures in Azerbaijan to seize additional territory, including the city of Agdam and surrounding towns (Croissant 1998). Armenian troops then advanced south to capture areas outside of Karabakh (Croissant 1998: 92). Around 350,000 Azeris were displaced by these new incursions, "one of the biggest refugee exoduses in Europe since the end of World War II" (de Waal

2013: 228). In desperation Azerbaijan requested refugee resettlement aid from the United Nations (Goltz 1998: 398). Armenia continued its advance and began targeting areas intended for Azerbaijan's oil pipeline construction, sending another 20,000 refugees across the nearby border into Iran (Croissant 1998: 93).

By the fall and winter of 1993 both sides accused one another of breaking cease fire agreements and the most intense phase of the conflict began. The Azeri army was now largely consolidated under Aliyev and reinforced by fighters from Afghanistan. Turkey supplied Azerbaijan with 150 military advisors and Russia provided 200 more (Croissant 1998: 96). These reinforced troops undertook a major offensive to reclaim territory north, south and east of Karabakh. Russian pilots were hired as mercenaries, even though they allegedly "had a habit of dropping bombs on Azeri cities just as peace was breaking out" (Goltz 1998: 434). Armenia received a good deal of support from its extensive diaspora community as well as from Russia. Late in 1993 Armenia pushed southward propelling thousands more Azeri villagers across the Araks River into Iran (de Waal 2013: 239). Fighting raged until the spring of 1994, when a peace agreement was brokered in Bishkek, Kyrgyzstan.

After the cease fire in 1994 a line of contact was established and the Republic of Artsakh was formed. This was a new territorial configuration, not recognized by Azerbaijan but under control of Armenia. No peacekeeping patrol was established, however, and both countries occupied the line with forces. Attempts to resolve the conflict stalled and the region became embedded in one of many "frozen" post-Soviet conflicts (Lachert 2019).

A map of the spatial distribution of confirmed conflicts between 1988–1994 shows that fighting occurred mostly around the mountainous NGK region (Fig. 3.1a). Conflicts were especially prevalent in the northern and eastern rayons. However, there were significant conflict sites outside of this area, particularly along the northern borders with Azerbaijan and Georgia, which were close to strategic energy pipeline corridors. Other battles occurred in regions south of NGK which is an important corridor along the Iranian border (Fig. 3.1a). Beginning in 1992, heavy fighting was occurring in Kalbajar, Agdam and Tartar rayons in the north and east of NGK. This led to hundreds of thousands of residents fleeing these areas (Fig. 3.1a).

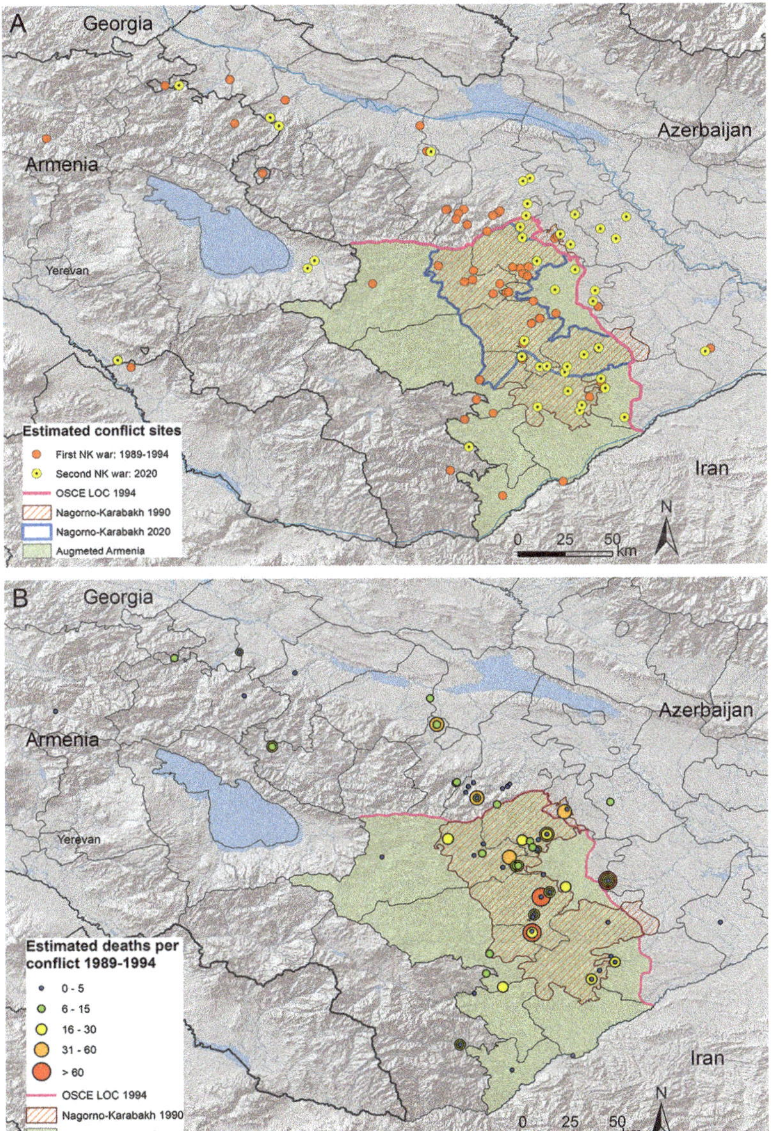


**Fig. 3.1** (a and b) South Caucasus region highlighting the estimated locations of known conflict sites and deaths during the Karabakh wars taken from the UCDP-PRIO dataset v22.1 (www.prio.org). (a) The approximate locations of conflict sites in Armenia and Azerbaijan from 1989–1994 (orange) and 2020 (yellow). (b) The estimated deaths per conflict site from 1989–1994. The historical Nagorno-Karabakh region (1990), the line of contact (LOC) from 1994. The Republic of Artsakh as well as the new Nagorno-Karabakh region (2020) are also indicated. Numerous conflict events per specific location occurred and therefore estimates per conflict event are stacked for some locations

Numerous conflict sites resulted in low estimates of casualties (Fig. 3.1b). However, there were many conflicts with high casualties, especially in the eastern regions of Nagorno-Karabakh and neighboring regions of Azerbaijan, including Agdam, Fuzuli and Tartar. Other conflict sites with large numbers of casualties occurred near the major cities of Stepanakert and Shusha, as well as in areas in the southeast of NGK bordering Iran (Fig. 3.1). Some of these areas are predominantly agricultural with a high density of villages.

Over 600 thousand ethnic Azeri IDPs from regions in and around NGK were displaced to cities, regions and/or settlement camps in Azerbaijan by the end of 1994 (UNHCR 2009). Most of these IDPs were settled in and around Baku, however, many others settled in one of several IDP camps facilitated by humanitarian organizations (UNHCR 2009). Additionally, several hundred thousand ethnic Armenians living in Azerbaijan were displaced by the end of 1994 (UNHCR 2008). As Armenia regained control of many areas around NK in 1994, many displaced ethnic Armenians from regions east of NGK, Baku, and Sumgait in Azerbaijan, slowly began to return to NGK and surrounding provinces (UNHCR 2008).

Since 1994, several resettlements of IDP in Azerbaijan have occurred (UNHCR 2009). In the early 1990s many camps and other improvised settlements were located far from the conflict in areas with different environmental and agricultural settings. In addition to being unfamiliar topography, these areas placed these populations in vulnerable health and economic conditions (UNHCR 2009). As a result of the resettlements that began in 2003 many IDPs relocated to areas closer to NGK, including Ganja, Agdam and Fuzuli. A geospatial analysis of IDPs in Fig. 3.2, shows the concentration of IDPs in regions to the east and south of NGK as of the mid-2000s. This placed IDPs into areas that more closely resembled their place of living prior to the conflict. The government of Azerbaijan in 2008 estimated that provinces surrounding NK, including Lachin, Agdam, Ganja and Fuzuli had nearly 160 thousand IDP combined.

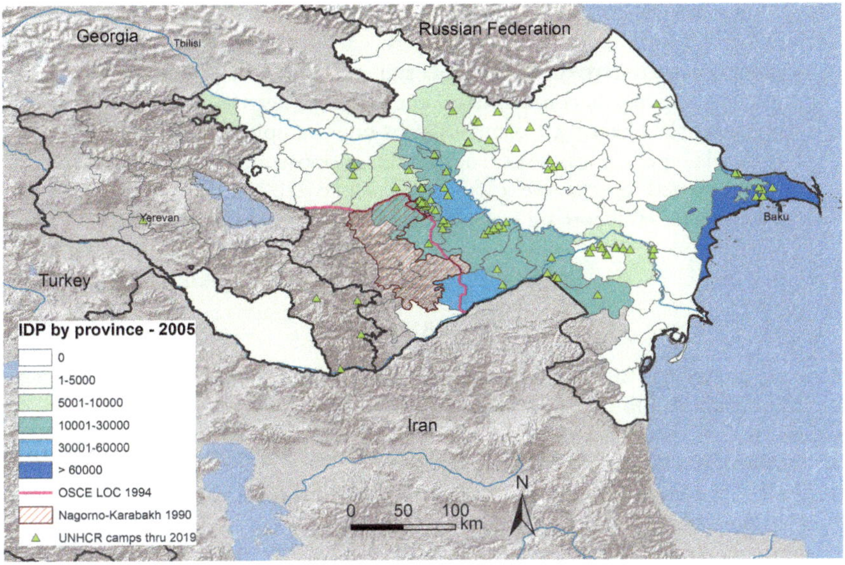


**Fig. 3.2** Overview of the South Caucasus showing the spatial distribution of UNHCR settlement camps and internally displaced persons (IDPs) by rayon in Azerbaijan as of 2005, according to reports from the Azerbaijan government and UNHCR. The historical Nagorno-Karabakh region (1990), the line of contact (LOC) from 1994, as well as the new Nagorno-Karabakh region (2020) are also indicated

## Notes

1. The Armenian genocide began in 1915. Much of the early violence was directed against Armenian enclaves in Ottoman Turkey. During World War I extreme nationalism led to more intense persecution of Armenians. Hundreds of families were placed in detention centers and Armenian cultural institutions (including churches) were targeted for destruction. There was also extensive plunder of Armenian property described by one scholar as "a state directed process ... closely linked to the development ... of the Armenian genocide" (Kurt 2018). It is estimated that between 800,000 and 1.5 million Armenians were killed between 1915 and 1922 (Demirdjian 2018).
2. It is likely that similar conditions prevailed in Azerbaijan during this time, but there are fewer written accounts available.

3. In the introduction to his memorable book on the Karabakh conflict, journalist Thomas Goltz described Azerbaijan as "doubly cursed" with "two greatest corrupters known to modern man: war and oil." He described how certain Azerbaijani commanders kept bodies of dead soldiers in refrigerators in order to collect their combat pay as one example of wartime corruption. But this type of wartime corruption was supposedly dwarfed by the corruption created by massive offshore oil discoveries. In 1991 the value of Azerbaijan's offshore oil was estimated at approximately $50 billion (Goltz 1998: xix).

## References


Broers, Laurence. 2021. *Armenia and Azerbaijan: Anatomy of a Rivalry.* Edinburgh: Edinburgh University Press.

Croissant, Michael. 1998. *The Armenia-Azerbaijan Conflict: Causes and Implications.* Westport, CT: Praeger.

de Waal, Thomas. 2013. *Black Garden: Armenia and Azerbaijan Through Peace and War.* New York: New York University Press.

Demirdjian, Alexis. 2018. The Turkish State and the Armenian Genocide. *Journal of International Criminal Justice*, 16: 501–526.

Dudwick, Nora. 1997. Political Transformation in Post-communist Armenia: Images and Realities. In *Conflict, Cleavage and Change in Central Asia and the Caucasus*, ed. Karen Dawisha and Bruce Parrott, 69–109. Cambridge: Cambridge University Press.

Goltz, Thomas. 1998. *Azerbaijan Diary.* Armonk, NY: M.E. Sharpe.

Horizon. 2019. Aliyev Admits Azerbaijan Worked to Boost Number of Azeris in Artsakh. https://horizonweekly.ca/en/aliyev-admits-azerbaijan-worked-to-boost-number-of-azerisin-artsakh/. Accessed March 2021.

Internal Displacement Monitoring Centre (IDMC). 2020. Global Report on Internal Displacement. https://www.internal-displacement.org/global-report/grid2020/. Accessed 30 October 2022.

Isaryan, Drastamat. 1994. Armenia: Until There Are No More Trees. *Bulletin of the Atomic Scientists* 50 (1): 28–31.

Kaldor, Mary. 2007. Oil and Conflict: The Case of Nagorno-Karabakh. In *Oil Wars*, ed. Mary Kaldor, Terry Lynn Karl, and Yahia Said, 157–182. London: Pluto Press.

Koehler, Jan, and Christoph Zurcher. 2003. The Art of Losing the State: Weak Empire to Weak Nation-State Around Nagorno-Karabakh. In *Potentials of Disorder: New Approaches to Conflict Analysis*, ed. Jan Koehler and Christoph Zurcher, 145–173. Manchester: Manchester University Press.

Kurt, Ümit. 2018. The Political Economy of the Armenian Genocide, 1915–1922. *Journal of Balkan and Near Eastern Studies*, 20(6): 618–638.

Lachert, Jakub. 2019. *Post-Soviet Frozen Conflicts: A Challenge for European Security*. Warsaw Institute. https://warsawinstitute.org/post-soviet-frozen-conflicts-challenge-europeansecurity/. Accessed 16 September 2022.

Los Angeles Times. July 20, 1993.

Mandic, Danilo. 2021. *Gangsters and Other Statesmen*. Princeton: Princeton University Press.

Marshall, Rick. 1993. *USAID Response to Armenian Situation*. Retrieved from RG 0268 Records of the United States Agency for International Development, National Archives and Records Administration, College Park, Maryland.

Nagorno Karabakh (NGK) Census. 2005. Table 1.3. Changes in the Numbers of De facto and De jure Population (Urban, Rural) of Nagorno-Karabakh by Sex, According to the Data of 1959, 1970, 1979, 1989, 2005 Censuses.. http://census.stat-nkr.am/nkr/1-3.pdf. Accessed April 2021.

UNHCR Report. 2008. Armenia: Analysis of Gaps in the Protection of Refugees and Asylum Seekers. UN High Commission for Refugees (UNHCR). https://www.ohchr.org/sites/default/files/lib-docs/HRBodies/UPR/Documents/Session8/AM/UNCTA_UPR_ARM_S08_2010_UNCountryTeamArmenia_Document4.pdf.

———. 2009. Azerbaijan: Analysis of Gaps in the Protection of Internally Displaced Persons (IDPs). UN High Commission for Refugees (UNHCR). https://www.unhcr.org/protection/convention/4bd7edbd9/azerbaijan-analysis-gaps-protection-internally-displaced-persons-idps.html.

Vartain, Ross. 1991. *Quarterly Progress Report from USAID Grantee Armenia Consortium to Tom Kirby, Consortium Program Manager, Project Hope*. September 30. Retrieved from RG 0268 Records of the United States Agency for International Development, National Archives and Records Administration, College Park, Maryland.

Zurcher, Christoph. 2007. *The Post-Soviet Wars: Rebellion, Ethnic Conflict and Nationhood in the Caucasus*. New York: NYU Press.

CHAPTER 4

# Rebordering, Forced Migration and Population Health Crises, 1988–1994

**Abstract** This chapter explores the population health crises that emerged as a result of the Karabakh conflict in the early 1990s. In addition to malaria, Armenia endured epidemics of measles, diphtheria, hepatitis and tuberculosis during this conflict. Most public services (including public health) collapsed after the disintegration of the USSR. The uncertainty of geopolitical boundaries during the conflict meant that some areas endured prolonged conditions of statelessness and "rebordering" that led to abandoned farmland, interruptions in agricultural production and massive population dislocations. Thousands of refugees were housed in poorly equipped camps for years while the conflict expanded. These conditions created tremendous vulnerability to epidemics of infectious disease.

**Keywords** Malaria • Rebordering • Armed conflict • Forced migration

The 1994 peace accord was fragile, but the cessation of hostilities allowed civilians and demobilized soldiers to exit combat zones and find shelter in refugee camps and urban settlements. Preliminary efforts were made to assess the war damage, including the loss of lives and destruction of agriculture and industry. According to one estimate approximately 25,000 people were killed or missing in combat (Broers 2021: 38). Official tallies are misleading, however, because there was never a clear line between formal armies, informal militias and civilians (Zurcher 2007). While the



K. Hirschfeld et al., *New Wars and Old Plagues*,
https://doi.org/10.1007/978-3-031-31143-7_4

overall number of conflict deaths in Karabakh was smaller than in the Bosnian or Chechen wars, the number of internally displaced persons (IDPs) was significantly higher (King 2008).

## 4.1 Rebordering and Forced Migration

The OSCE line of contact was established to demarcate the de facto Republic of Artsakh, which was formed after the 1994 conflict (see Fig. 3.1b). It consisted of NGK and the surrounding territory reaching to the borders of Iran in the south and Armenia in the west. This territorial configuration represents one potential iteration of "augmented Armenia," the vision of ancestral territorial claims developed by some Armenian nationalists after the cease fire agreement in 1994 (Broers 2021). Augmented Armenia includes seven districts surrounding NGK that were previously part of Azerbaijan. As Broers described, these additional territories "comprised more than the original surface area of the NKAO's 4,400 square kilometers" (Broers 2021: 98). This expanded cartography was incorporated into the Armenian body politic and many Azeri place names were changed to evoke Armenia's "medieval geographies" (Broers 2021). Broers goes on to state that the idea of augmented Armenia is "problematic because it combines the legitimacy of self-determination with the illegitimacy of occupation and ethnic cleansing" (2021: 102).

Azerbaijan was more internally fragmented than Armenia after the Soviet collapse, and there was no immediate national consensus on the territorial claims surrounding the Karabakh conflict. But over time a competing vision of "wider Azerbaijan" emerged and its national vision absorbed all of present-day Armenia. As Broers described,

> [Wide Azerbaijan] is a geopolitical vision that absorbs a modern Armenian territoriality in its entirety. Its implications are obvious: a historically deepened and horizontally elongated Azerbaijan edges Armenia out of the Caucasus ... Whereas Armenian practices trace their palimpsest across large swathes of western Azerbaijan, Azerbaijan's is more total in extending over all of Armenia. Contemporary Azerbaijani textbooks depict early nineteenth-century Azerbaijan as a wide, homogenous geo-body stretching from the Caspian to Igdir in the west. (2021: 118)

Azerbaijan's ethnonationalism also led to mass expulsion of Armenian citizens from its body politic during the early phase of conflict. Over

500,000 ethnic Armenians lived in Baku before the war. By 1995 only about 10,000 remained (Goltz 1998: xxii). Due to the food and energy crisis in Armenia, an estimated 667,000 Armenians fled the country to live abroad, with slightly less than half coming from the city of Yerevan itself. Armenia lost 18% of its population to outmigration, and the capital city lost nearly 25% of its inhabitants (Dudwick 1997: 83). Over 80,000 Armenian refugees were still living in camps many years after the 1994 peace accord was signed, and "hundreds of thousands more were living in a vast archipelago of sanatoria, student hostels and makeshift accommodations" (de Waal 2013: 230).

Conflict-driven population movements have been undertheorized by social scientists. As Danilo Mandic has noted, "Unforced migrants ... dominate the theoretical agenda" of migration studies (2022: 61). But recent work in political sociology has better framed forced population movements as part of the violent identity politics characteristic of New Wars. One key element of this updated social theory is the explicit delineation of one or more "force factors" displacing multitudes of people in a relatively compressed time span. Force factors include varieties of "violent social actors" including militias, organized crime groups, warlords, nation-state armies and revolutionary movements (Mandic 2022).

Several scholars have detailed how these violent expulsions have become common in New War conflicts (Broers 2021; Kaldor 2012; Malesevic 2010). Russia's 2022 invasion of Ukraine, for instance, produced an unprecedented wave of forced depopulation intended to pave the way for Russian occupation. Over 7 million refugees exited the country within the first few months of fighting due to the extreme violence targeting civilians and civilian infrastructure (UNHCR.org/en/situationsukraine). Similarly destructive conflicts have also been waged in Syria, Iraq, Afghanistan and Yemen. In the Western hemisphere the Cartel zones in Mexico and Central America continue to displace an estimated 400,000 people per year due to "environmental challenges and chronic violence" (Cheatham and Roy 2022).

These forced population movements create massive vulnerabilities to infectious disease outbreaks, as IDPs abandon their homesteads and relocate to crowded refugee camps or improvised housing. When political space is contested for long periods of time public health surveillance and vector control efforts are disrupted or abandoned. Preventable diseases can re-emerge and circulate undetected in these spaces until order is re-established or afflicted populations migrate to areas that have operational

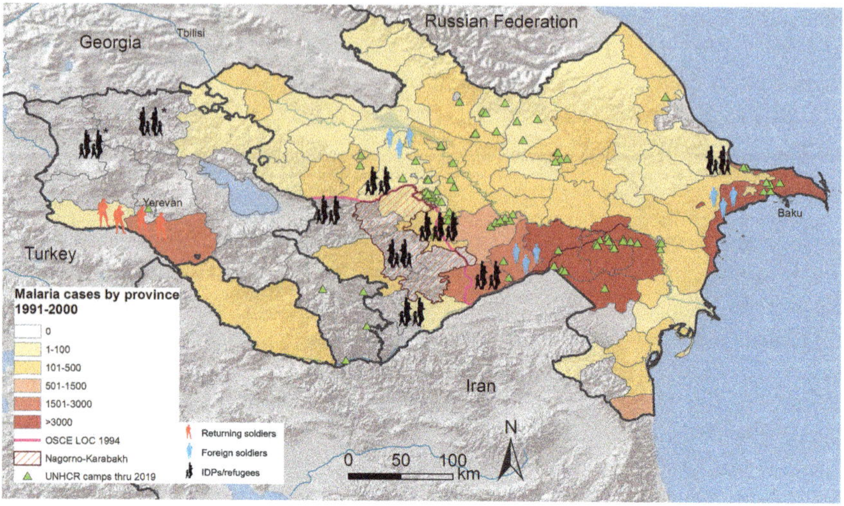


**Fig. 4.1** Geographic overview of violence, population displacement and documented malaria cases (1991–1998) during the Karabakh conflict. The position, level and direction of IDP/refugee movement as well as returning soldier position are best estimates based on relevant literature

health infrastructure and resources to detect outbreaks. When armed conflicts are centered in rural areas, population movements can have major impacts on agricultural production and lead to widespread abandonment of croplands. Abandoned croplands—especially those fed by irrigation canals—create ideal breeding grounds for anopheles mosquitoes. Outbreaks can also follow impoverished migrants fleeing conflict zones, and foreign mercenary fighters or peacekeepers coming into conflict zones (Katz 2016). These dynamics are all visible in Fig. 4.1, which details the spatial distribution of displaced persons, violence and malaria cases during the most intense phase of the Karabakh conflict.

## 4.2 Forced Migration and Population Health Crises

In addition to the forced expulsion of hundreds of thousands of Armenians and Azeris during the conflict, new populations of foreign soldiers were brought into the region. While both sides had foreign fighters, Azerbaijan seemed to recruit more of them, including an estimated 1500–2000 mujahideen from Afghanistan soon after Aliyev took power (Taarnby 2008; de Waal 2013; Goltz 1998). Documents and materials found on the battlefield support this, including notes on armory positions, tactics and instructions, photos and personal letters, all in Pashto (Sneider 1993). Captured soldiers and Armenian Ministry of Defense reports also suggest that the Azerbaijan government actively arranged recruiting, housing and training in Azerbaijan, with the help of Russian and US citizens (Taarnby 2008; Goltz 1998).

During the 1970s and 1980s Afghanistan had high rates of malaria and reported several hundred thousand cases annually (WHO 1999). It is estimated that millions of malaria cases occurred in Afghanistan in the early 1990s (WHO 1998). The ability of *P. vivax* to lay dormant in the human body for months increases the potential for introduction of malaria into conflict zones. Population dislocations amplified outbreaks of infectious disease throughout the conflict, especially in landlocked Armenia where it became almost impossible to import food and essential medical supplies. In 1992 inflation reached approximately 360% per year and food supplies were scarce. A December 1992 cable from the US Embassy in Yerevan noted the country had little to no supply of surgical anesthesia, infant formula or milk. Infant mortality was predicted to rise and "diseases associated with contaminated water and standing sewerage, and malnutrition are anticipated" (USAID 1992).

After the devastating earthquake in 1988, a team of international aid workers supported by USAID was permitted by the USSR to engage in humanitarian relief work in Armenia. Many of the medical professionals on this mission were specialists in reconstructive surgery and rehabilitation. But as living conditions worsened additional teams were sent to Armenia including epidemiologists and emergency medicine specialists. One visiting surgeon described his working conditions in the winter of 1993 as follows,

> This quarter coincided with serious disruptions and worsening of overall conditions in Armenia. The winter was the worst in over thirty years. Economic problems were profound. Public transportation was virtually nonexistent much of the time. Prices for food and staples were increasing at double digit inflationary rates. Electricity throughout the country was reduced to 1-2 hours per day maximum with many people without electricity (and water) for days. All morbidity/mortality rates for all age groups rose

> dramatically. People starved to death and froze to death within hospitals in Yerevan. Most of the city of Yerevan hospitals and clinics closed, as did rural clinics and policlinics. (McIntyre 1993)

The black market price of gasoline was reported by the *New York Times* to be 7500 rubles for 5 gallons, twice the average monthly salary. Desperate for heat during the freezing winter months, Armenians cut down trees in Karabakh, as well as in urban and rural areas all over the country (*New York Times*, February 7, 1993). In December 1992 a State Department Cable described the growing crisis as follows,

> A national emergency exists in Armenia. Armenia faces the prospect of disintegration, catastrophic hardship and starvation of the small, weak and infirm ... The blockade has effectively ended any substantive importation of fuel and curtailed imports of food required by Armenians ... Until the blockade is lifted, broken or modified to allow the importation of food and fuel, Armenia will require continual humanitarian assistance and support. All major industry is closed. There is no continuing supply of natural gas. Extended power blackouts are affecting all sections of Yerevan ... By late December there will be no milk or baby formula in country ... 597,000 elderly Armenian pensioners also require food supplements ... The blockade has also left Armenia without medical reserves. (USAID 1992)

A team of epidemiologists from the Centers for Disease Control in Atlanta was dispatched to Armenia work with local public health professionals and rebuild disease surveillance capabilities (Balasanian and McNabb 2000; McNabb et al. 1994; Wuhib et al. 2002). These groups collaborated on a population health census that revealed alarming trends. Almost 90% of elderly residents were found to be experiencing severe poverty and hunger. Monthly rates of measles increased by 60% since the 1980s, diarrheal illness by 61%, viral hepatitis by 163% and tuberculosis by 75% (USAID 1992). Diphtheria was spreading in rural and urban areas. Based on the CDC assessments, US government agencies predicted up to 30,000 deaths from starvation unless additional food assistance was provided to Armenia. US State Department cables also described a total refugee population in Armenia of over 400,000 with approximately 100,000 people living in "sub-human conditions" (UNHCR telegram from Yerevan to Multiple US Agencies and Embassies, September 1992).

## 4.3 Resurgent Malaria and Environmental Change

The first cases of malaria recognized in Armenia during the Karabakh conflict were almost all imported, with one locally acquired or autochthonous case identified in 1994. Another 502 imported cases were recorded in 1995, with most in Masis district south of Yerevan (Avetisyan 2002; Davidyants et al. 2019). The epidemic peaked in 1998, with 1156 total cases reported, with 89% in the villages of the Masis district (Davidyants et al. 2019). This pattern suggested a local introduction which facilitated malaria re-emergence in this region of Armenia.

Returning soldiers and displaced persons would have been susceptible during fighting on the front lines as surveillance and control measures were disrupted. Conflicts were heavy in the areas east and south of NGK, especially in 1993, with thousands of displaced people and extensive land abandonment (Fig. 3.2). These areas are also significantly lower in elevation and possess extensive agriculture and irrigation, as compared to the mountainous NGK region. An outbreak of malaria also developed in Azerbaijan beginning soon afterward, predominantly in the central and southern river valleys (Mammadov et al. 2016).

The influx of foreign mercenaries from malaria-endemic regions such as Afghanistan most likely reintroduced *P. vivax* to the Caucasus, though it is difficult to be certain without more thorough epidemiological research.[1] The rapid concentration of displaced persons in improvised housing and refugee camps in lowland areas provided a large pool of vulnerable human hosts to fuel an expanding epidemic. During the conflict period, the Ministries of Health were unable to conduct routine mosquito surveillance and chemical abatement procedures as they had done previously (Wuhib et al. 2002). As a result, mosquito populations previously under control were largely untouched throughout the lowland agricultural areas of Armenia and Azerbaijan. *Anopheles sacharovi*, the most common vector for malaria in the region reappeared after the conflict (Boccolini et al. 2000; Romi et al. 2002; Severini et al. 2004). Cases of malaria peaked in 1996 and 1998, respectively (Fig. 4.2). Figure 4.2 shows the accumulated cases of malaria from 1994–1999 in the provinces of Armenia and Azerbaijan. In Armenia, cases began to appear in 1994 in the population centers south of Yerevan in the provinces of Ararat and Armavir, all within the agriculturally productive Araks River valley (CDC 1998; Avetisyan 2002; Davidvants et al. 2019).

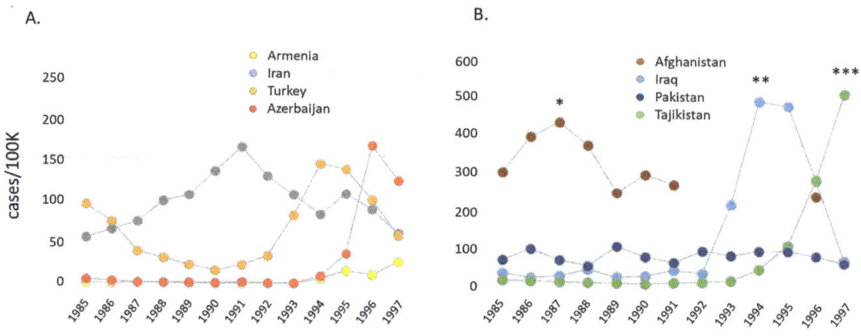


**Fig. 4.2** (a) Malaria cases per 100K population of malaria from 1985 through 1997 in the Caucasus and neighboring countries (b) in other regional conflict zones. Cases of malaria are taken from the WHO World Epidemiological Reports. *peak of malaria during the conflict between Afghanistan and the Soviet Union. **peak of malaria after the first Iraq-US Persian Gulf war. ***increase in malaria cases in Tajikistan following the start of civil war

At the beginning of the outbreak in 1994 and 1995, more than 90% of cases occurred in displaced persons and soldiers returning from the conflict areas around NK (CDC 1998; Avetisyan 2002). IDPs from the NGK region may have been more susceptible to malaria infection due to lack of immunity as NGK is more protected from malaria than other areas due to its elevation (Avetisyan 2002). Furthermore, their placement in makeshift camps in lowland regions highly susceptible to malaria would have put them at increased risk for exposure (see Fig. 3.2). While the numbers of cases of malaria in these UNHCR camps were not available they were located in heavily irrigated lowland areas, prone to malaria (Mammadov et al. 2016; Bruce-Chwatt 1959). Indeed, UNHCR reports suggest that malaria control measures were implemented in the late 1990s in many of these camps, including anti-malarial drugs, insecticidal spraying and bed net distribution (UNHCR Report 2009). The nature of the settlement camp infrastructure and condition in combination with its location likely increased the chances of malaria outbreaks.

Over 90% of Armenia's locally acquired cases in 1996 were from three cities in the provinces south of Yerevan: Masis, Vedi and Artashat (Avetisyan 2002). This suggests that widespread transmission was only occurring in this area. In Azerbaijan, most malaria cases occurred in the provinces to the east of NGK in the lowlands of the Kura River valley and in provinces along the Araks River bordering Iran (Mammadov et al. 2016; Avetisyan

2002; CDC 1998; Temel 2007). These areas to the south of Yerevan and in the south and west of Azerbaijan are regions of high agricultural productivity. Regionally, there were also increases in malaria cases in Iran, Iraq and Turkey as well during the early 1990s, as detailed in Fig. 4.2. In Turkey, increases in malaria were largely due to construction of the Southeastern Anatolia Irrigation Project or GAP in the early 1990s (Askoy et al. 1995).

Armenia's geographical location supports several distinct anopheles mosquito populations, including those from the southern and eastern Mediterranean, Middle East and Central Asia. Recent reports have also suggested that mosquito population dynamics and *Plasmodium* parasite biology have changed since the 1970s, including those found in Armenia (Romi et al. 2002; Kondrashin et al. 2018). Increases in the number of reactivated *P. vivax* cases or long-term cases of malaria have also been observed in many areas of Russia, Central Asia and the Caucasus (Kondrashin et al. 2018). These changes have the potential to facilitate the re-emergence of malaria in these regions, especially if conflict and political instability return.

There is no vaccine for *P. vivax* malaria, and (as detailed in Chap. 2) malaria eradication in the Caucasus during the twentieth century took decades of sustained authoritarian measures. *P. vivax* is especially challenging to control since it can remain dormant in the human body during winter months and re-emerge in the spring when mosquitoes begin to hatch. Furthermore, *P. vivax* can be asymptomatic in a host with some immunity and regular exposure but create devastating epidemics in immunologically naive populations. Successful control of malaria requires multiple interventions including modifications of the landscape to eliminate standing water or seasonal flooding, use of insecticides to reduce mosquito populations and regular dosing of susceptible human populations with anti-malarial drugs. Unfortunately, remote sensing research shows that even short periods of armed conflict can reshape the landscape in ways that facilitate expanded breeding sites for anopheles mosquitoes.

## Note

1. Azerbaijan was known to have malaria outbreaks in the 1980s and 1990s and disease surveillance near the conflict zone was quite poor. So it is also possible that malaria was introduced by Azeri troops rather than Afghani fighters.

## References

Askoy, Serap, Sedat Ariturk, Martine Y.K. Armstrong, K.P. Chang, Zeynep Dörtbudak, Gottleib Michael, M. Ali Ozcel, Frank F. Richards, and Karl Western. 1995. The GAP Project in Southeastern Turkey: The Potential for Emergence of Diseases. *Emerging Infectious Diseases* 1 (2): 62–63.

Avetisyan, Lilit. 2002. Re-emergence of Malaria in Armenia and Vector Control Interventions. *Journal of Health Sciences Management and Public Health*. https://pdfs.semanticscholar.org/36f4/73779a798015b70c270d6b52769cfefeb88d.pdf. Accessed 4 September 2020.

Balasanian, Margarita, and Scott J.N. McNabb. 2000. Epidemic Investigation of Diphtheria in the Republic of Armenia, 1990–1996. *Journal of Infectious Disease* 181 (Suppl 1): S69–S72.

Boccolini, Daniela, Roberto Romi, Marco Di Luca, I. Hovanesyan, G. Grigoryan, Giancarlo Majori, and Guido Sabatinelli. 2000. Entomological Investigations on the Malaria Epidemic in Armenia: Role of *Anopheles sacharovi*. *Parassitologia* 42 (Suppl 1): 124.

Broers, Laurence. 2021. *Armenia and Azerbaijan: Anatomy of a Rivalry*. Edinburgh: Edinburgh University Press.

Bruce-Chwatt, Leonard J. 1959. Malaria Research and Eradication in the USSR: A Review of Soviet Achievements in the Field of Malariology. *Bulletin of the World Health Organization* 21: 737–772.

Centers for Disease Control (CDC). 1998. Epidemic Malaria Transmission in Armenia, 1997. *Morbidity and Mortality Weekly Report*. https://www.cdc.gov/mmwr/preview/mmwrhtml/00053695.htm. Accessed 4 September 2020.

Cheatham, Amelia, and Roy, Diana. 2022. Central America's Turbulent Northern Triangle. Council on Foreign Relations. https://www.cfr.org/backgrounder/central-americasturbulent-northern-triangle. Accessed 11 September 2022.

Davidyants, Vladimir A., Anatoly V. Kondrashin, Artavazd V. Vanyan, Lola F. Morozova, Natalia A. Turbabina, Ekaterina V. Stepanova, Maria S. Maksimova, and Evgeny N. Morozov. 2019. Role of Malaria Partners in Malaria Elimination in Armenia. *Malaria Journal* May 22; 18(1): 178. https://doi.org/10.1186/s12936-019-2814-y.

de Waal, Thomas. 2013. *Black Garden: Armenia and Azerbaijan Through Peace and War*. New York: New York University Press.

Dudwick, Nora. 1997. Political Transformation in Post-communist Armenia: Images and Realities. In *Conflict, Cleavage and Change in Central Asia and the Caucasus*, ed. Karen Dawisha and Bruce Parrott, 69–109. Cambridge: Cambridge University Press.

Goltz, Thomas. 1998. *Azerbaijan Diary*. Armonk, NY: M.E. Sharpe.

Internal Displacement Monitoring Centre (IDMC). 2020. Global Report on Internal Displacement. https://www.internal-displacement.org/global-report/grid2020/. Accessed 30 October 2022.

Kaldor, Mary. 2012. *Old and New Wars.* Malden, MA: Polity Press.

Katz, Jonathan. 2016. UN Admits Role in Cholera Epidemic in Haiti. *New York Times.* https://www.nytimes.com/2016/08/18/world/americas/united-nations-haiti-cholera.html. Accessed 11 September 2022.

King, Charles. 2008. *The Ghost of Freedom: A History of the Caucasus.* Oxford: Oxford University Press.

Kondrashin, A. V., L. F. Morozova, E. V. Stepanova, N. A. Turbabina, M. S. Maksimova, and E. N. Morozov. 2018. On the epidemiology of Plasmodium vivax malaria: past and present with special reference to the former USSR. *Malaria Journal* 17 (1): 346.

Malesevic, Sinisa. 2010. *The Sociology of War and Violence.* Cambridge: Cambridge University Press.

Mammadov, Suleyman, Elkhan Gasimov, Rossitza Kurdova-Mintcherva, and Chansuda Wongsrichanalai. 2016. Elimination of *Plasmodium vivax* Malaria in Azerbaijan. *American Journal of Tropical Medicine Hygiene* 95 (Suppl 6): 78–86.

Mandic, Danilo. 2022. What Is the Force Is Forced Migration? *Theory and Society* 51: 61–90. https://link.springer.com/article/10.1007/s11186-021-09446-0/. Accessed 10 November 2022.

McIntyre, Michael. 1993. *Quarterly Report Filed from Armenia. United States Agency for International Development, January–March.* Retrieved from RG 0286 Records of the United States Agency for International Development. National Archives and Records Administration, College Park, Maryland.

McNabb, Scott J., Kathleen Welch, Sandy Laumark, Dan E. Peterson, Raoult C. Ratard, Michael J. Toole, and Thomas A. Farley. 1994. Population-based Nutritional Risk Survey of Pensioners in Yerevan, Armenia. *American Journal of Preventative Medicine* 10 (2): 65–70.

Romi, Roberto, Daniela Boccolini, I. Hovanesyan, G. Grigoryan, Marco Di Luca, and Guido Sabatinelli. 2002. *Anopheles sacharovi* (Diptera: Culicidae): A Reemerging Malaria Vector in the Ararat Valley of Armenia. *Journal of Medical Entomology* 39 (3): 446–450.

Severini, Francesco, Marco Di Luca, Carlo Severini, Vladimir Davidyants, Lilit Avetisyan, Roberto Romi, and Giancarlo Majori. 2004. Malaria Surveillance Activities in Armenia: Results of an Entomological Survey. *Parassitologia* 46 (Suppl 1): 101.

Sneider, Daniel. 1993. Afghan Fighters Join Azeri-Armenian War. *Christian Science Monitor.* November 16, 1993. https://www.csmonitor.com/1993/1116/16071.html. Accessed 2 February 2020.

Taarnby, Michael. 2008. *The Mujahedin in Nagorno-Karabakh: A Case Study in the Evolution of Global Jihad.* The Real Institute El Cano (Elcano Royal Institute), Madrid, Spain.

Temel, Tugrul. 2007. Malaria from the Gap: Need for Cross-Sector Cooperation in Azerbaijan. *SSRN*. https://doi.org/10.2139/ssrn.986502.

UNHCR Report. 2009. Azerbaijan: Analysis of Gaps in the Protection of Internally Displaced Persons (IDPs). UN High Commission for Refugees (UNHCR). https://www.unhcr.org/protection/convention/4bd7edbd9/azerbaijan-analysis-gaps-protection-internally-displaced-persons-idps.html.

USAID. 1992. Unclassified Agency Telecommunications Yerevan December. Retrieved from RG 0268 Records of the United States Agency for International Development, National Archives and Records Administration, College Park, Maryland.

World Health Organization (WHO). 1998. Weekly Epidemiological Record. *World Health Organization* 73 (13): 89–96.

———. 1999. Weekly Epidemiological Record: Malaria, 1982–1997. August 13, 1999, 74: 265–272.

Wuhib, Tadesse, Terrence L. Chorba, Vladimir Davidyants, William R. MacKenzie, and Scott J. McNabb. 2002. Assessment of the Infectious Diseases Surveillance System of the Republic of Armenia: An Example of Surveillance in the Republics of the Former Soviet Union. *BMC Public Health* 2: 3.

Zurcher, Christoph. 2007. *The Post-Soviet Wars: Rebellion, Ethnic Conflict and Nationhood in the Caucasus*. New York: NYU Press.

CHAPTER 5

# Long-Term Conflict and Environmental Change

**Abstract** The Karabakh conflict reignited in the winter of 2020 and a new peace accord transferred several key regions from Armenian to Azeri control. At least 90,000 people were displaced and tensions in the region remain high. This chapter uses data from remote sensing to assess the long-term environmental impact of the Karabakh conflict from the 1990s through 2020. We look specifically at changes in land use and land cover. These include analyses of forest disturbance, cropland abandonment and patterns of surface water. We conclude that forest disturbance and cropland abandonment are likely to generate expanded habitat for *Anopheles sacharovi*—a key malaria vector in the region. Ongoing tensions also suggest the conflict is not yet resolved and the potential for new hostilities is high.

**Keywords** Deforestation • Cropland abandonment • Land use • Land cover

## 5.1 Resurgent Conflict and Rebordering, 2020

The 1994 cease fire agreement did not establish a peacekeeping patrol along the line of contact, and both countries occupied the line with forces. Low intensity violence was a regular feature in the region with dozens of people killed or injured in border skirmishes almost every year. In 2016 four days of fighting led to hundreds of deaths near the line of


K. Hirschfeld et al., *New Wars and Old Plagues*,
https://doi.org/10.1007/978-3-031-31143-7_5

demarcation (Crisis Group 2022a, 2022b). In a 2017 report, Thomas de Waal described the area transforming from "a string of hastily dug trenches separating the two armies" in 1994 to "the most militarized zone in Europe, bristling with artillery, long range missile launchers, attack helicopters and military drones" in 2017 (de Waal 2017).

Intense fighting erupted again in September 2020 and continued for approximately six weeks. By October, Azeri forces approached the Lachin Corridor and threatened Armenia's control of surrounding regions. In retaliation, Armenia launched an offensive along Azeri supply routes. Soon after, Azeri military forces surrounded the historic town of Shusha forcing Armenian inhabitants to flee to nearby Stepanakert. Days of intense street fighting followed with "building to building close combat" (Spencer and Ghoorhoo 2021).

Before fleeing the area, many Armenians intentionally set fire to their properties "finding solace in knowing their enemies could never sleep there" (Cookman 2020). They also killed their livestock or released their animals to roam free along high mountain roads. One reporter described witnessing a tragic "large scale migration of people from a land that … literally changed owners overnight." One reporter estimated that approximately 90,000 people had been displaced during the 2020 conflict out of a total of about 150,000 in the territory (Kucera 2020). The conflict once again left thousands of refugees stranded without communications, heat, hot water or adequate food. Displaced people expressed confusion, shock and uncertainty about where the new territorial boundaries were located (Cookman 2020).

In the 1980s, Shusha had been home to approximately 23,000 Azeri residents and the town had great symbolic importance as "the cradle of Azeri culture" (Spencer and Ghoorhoo 2021). Most of these residents were killed or forced into exile during the Armenian offensive in 1992. At that time the town was resettled by Armenians but remained underpopulated with only about 5000 inhabitants in 2020 (Spencer and Ghoorhoo 2021). By November the town was fully under Azeri military control and a "lopsided" peace deal was signed that transferred Armenian controlled areas surrounding Karabakh back to Azerbaijan (Spencer and Ghoorhoo 2021). More than 7000 casualties were reported, including soldiers and civilians. Hundreds more were wounded (Global Conflict Tracker 2022). An estimated 30,000 Armenians were forced out of their homes in the area on short notice (de Waal 2021).

The 2020 peace accord was brokered by Russia, and included an agreement that seven districts adjacent to Karabakh that were integrated into augmented Armenia after the 1994 cease fire would be returned to Azerbaijan. Karabakh lost substantially more of its croplands than the area that was recaptured by Azerbaijan. The area of augmented Armenia delineated after the 1994 cease fire was approximately 1683 km$^2$. The smaller area of Soviet era Nagorno-Karabakh was 4495 km$^2$, with 4262 km$^2$ within the line of contact after the cease fire of 1994. After the 2020 conflict, the remaining area of Karabakh was reduced to approximately 3259 km$^2$, shrinking the entire area under Armenian control by about 72% and shrinking Nagorno-Karabakh by about 24%.

Russian troops are scheduled to remain in place until 2025 to protect Azeri transit corridors between Karabakh and Armenia, as well as between the enclave of Nakhichevan and Azerbaijan (Sestanovich 2020). As detailed by Thomas de Waal, this accord "radically changes the geopolitical configuration of the region, giving Moscow a central role it last held in the Soviet era" (2021). De Waal goes on to state that the peace accord does not appear stable, with both countries continuing to act "as if they are still at war" (2021). Azerbaijan has allegedly resisted turning over Armenian captives and some Armenian forces remain in Karabakh due to uncertainty about the exact terms of the peace accord.

The revised 2020 territorial boundaries also create trade and transit problems. Much of the Karabakh region has been cut off from Armenia but is not yet integrated into the economy or polity of Azerbaijan. According to de Waal, Azerbaijan's President Aliyev "has indicated that he intends to keep up a policy of isolating Karabakh from the outside world and severing its political connections with Armenia" (2021). Armenia has also refused to surrender some land claimed by Azerbaijan, including seven villages in the Kazakh District (de Waal 2021). There have been reports of widespread destruction of Armenian churches, cemeteries and cultural monuments in the Nakhichevan region as well as in reclaimed areas of Karabakh (Isayev 2022; Maghakyan 2022; Nutt 2022).

These tensions led to new hostilities in the fall of 2022. Nearly 300 people were killed after Azerbaijan shelled several villages inside Armenia (Crisis Group 2022c). The shelling continued for two days along Armenia's eastern border until it was halted by a fragile cease fire with both sides accusing each other of instigating territorial aggression (Crisis Group 2022c). Both sides claimed to be unclear about where the actual border between the two countries currently falls. Several analysts have claimed that Russia's 2022 invasion of Ukraine has further destabilized the Karabakh region by distracting Russia's attention and revealing the extent of Russia's military weakness to leaders in Azerbaijan and Armenia (Glantz 2022). The threat of a new offensive has been described as "very high" and prospects for peace are looking "increasingly slim" (Crisis Group 2022c).

## 5.2 Long-Term Conflict and Environmental Change

The Karabakh region has endured more than 30 years of unresolved conflict and territorial instability with repeated rounds of rebordering, forced migration and resettlement. To assess the cumulative impact of these events on patterns of land use and land cover, we conducted an extensive geospatial analysis that included the following components: (1) a topographic analysis to measure elevation and wetness; (2) a cropland analysis to assess changes in land use and extent of croplands disturbed or abandoned during the conflict; (3) a forest disturbance analysis to assess the impact of the conflict on tree cover; (4) a brief analysis of land and village abandonment and how these factors may have increased mosquito breeding sites after the cessation of formal hostilities. This geographic analysis reveals that multiple environmental disturbances from the conflict changed the landscape in ways that created extensive habitat for *Anopheles sacharovi*—a key malaria vector in the region.

During times of armed conflict there are often a series of direct and indirect environmental consequences. Direct effects of conflicts can result from an increase in fires and clearcutting, such as was visible in the 2020 Karabakh conflict when 889 forest fires were recorded between October 22 and November 3 (ACAPS 2020). Indirect effects are often more subtle but can be longer lasting. One relevant example is the deforestation that took place in Armenia as a result of the energy embargo imposed by Azerbaijan during the 1990s. The energy crisis lasted several winters and Armenians cut thousands of trees as their source for heating.

In addition to changes in forests and croplands, surface water is another important aspect of the land which is relevant to this conflict and its associated epidemic of malaria. Water shortages and droughts are major sources of concern in Azerbaijan (Palazzo 2020). Several important water reservoirs are located on the recaptured lands, such as the large water reservoir in Mataghis which feeds water to the Sarsang water facility and is currently still controlled by Yerevan-backed separatists. Another reservoir in Mataghis is very important for the irrigation of croplands in the southern part of our study region. Before the 2020 conflict, the irrigation canal from Sarsang that fed these croplands was not providing water to Azerbaijani lowland croplands (Palazzo 2020). Abundant water from the mountainous regions fed large river systems for both Armenia and Azerbaijan.

Overall, our analysis reveals agricultural infrastructure sustained severe damage throughout the primary conflict region. An estimated 22 miles of irrigation channels, which provided water to more than 47,000 acres of farmland, were damaged or rendered dysfunctional due to the disabling of water reservoirs and pumping stations. Abandoned irrigation channels can easily get clogged causing salinization and fertilizer contamination. Disruptions in operations of these irrigation channels in these areas have the potential to create abundant mosquito habitat. While direct relationship between malaria and area of irrigated land is hard to pinpoint, the vast development of irrigated water in these arid regions is an important component for maintaining mosquito density. Populations in and around these areas, including IDPs would be under increased potential for malaria and other vector borne diseases if left unmaintained and abatement procedures were not implemented.

The croplands in post-configuration 2020 Nagorno-Karabakh are generally found on higher elevations, with steeper slopes and low topographic water indices, making these areas less suitable for cultivation than the croplands within the recaptured area. In addition, there was minimal forest loss in both regions ($<30\text{km}^2$ per year), but major forest disturbance, which can represent forest thinning or other damage (approximately $200\text{km}^2$ appears disturbed in the combined region). Additional forest disturbance occurred in the summer of 2020. Since satellite images were recorded before the conflict (June–August 2020), this is most likely not related to the fighting that occurred in the fall. A substantial increase in the number of fires—889 vs approximately 90 in previous years—was detected in the region as a direct result of the conflict. Impacts of these fires should be visible in disturbance data from 2021 (ACAPS 2020).

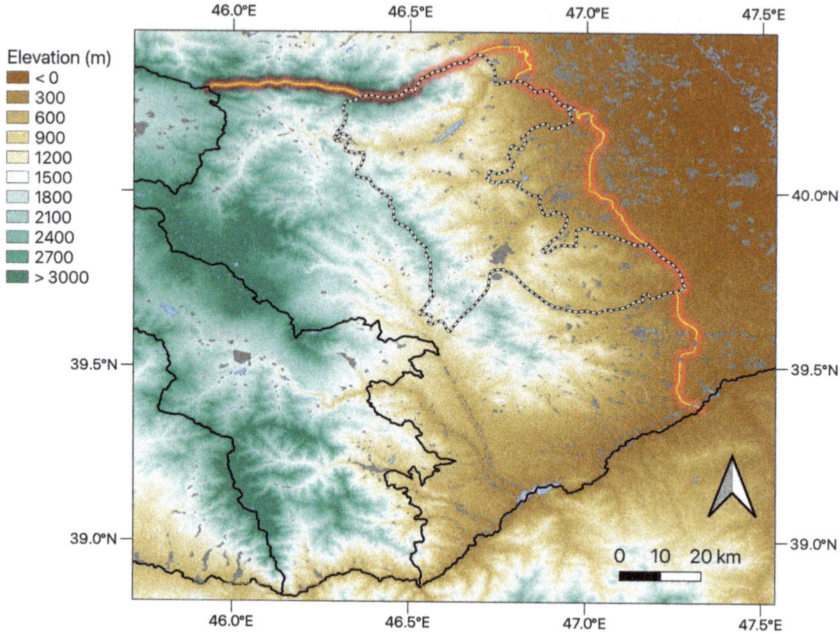


**Fig. 5.1** The digital elevation model reveals that most areas of 1994 era Greater Karabakh/augmented Armenia are highly elevated, with the highest elevations in the West along the border with Armenia. There are lowland areas in the southern part along the border with Iran. Urban areas are gray

## 5.3 Topographic Analysis

The average and median elevations for the 1994 era greater Karabakh/ augmented Armenia (which Armenians call Artsakh) are 1277m and 1105m respectively (Fig. 5.1). The average and median slopes are 12.5° and 11.2° (Fig. 5.2A, top). This mountainous area only has some gentler slopes in the southern part on the border with Iran and in the eastern part near Stepanakert/Khankendi. The average elevation of the post-reconfiguration 2020 Nagorno-Karabakh region (PR-2020) is a bit lower, 1119m for the mean elevation and 1026m for the median elevation, but the slopes for PR-2020 are steeper than the overall slopes: the mean slope is 13.9° and the median slope is 12.9°.

Figure 5.1 depicts the slopes for 1994 era greater Karabakh/augmented Armenia and PR-2020. Only the most southern part of the 1994 era greater Karabakh/augmented Armenia has gentle slopes, as well as some

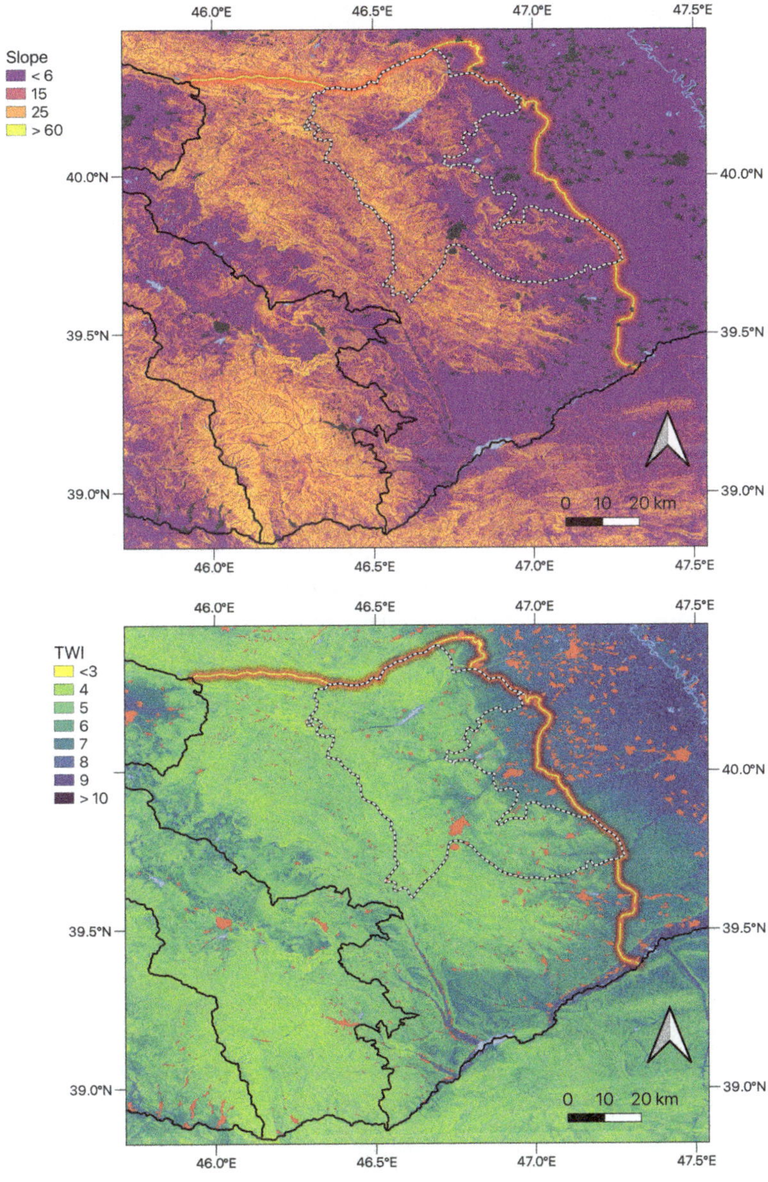


**Fig. 5.2** A (top) and B (bottom) The slope (top) and the topographic wetness index (bottom) show that only the far southern area of 1994 era Greater Karabakh/augmented Armenia has suitable slopes (<6°) for croplands. Those areas are also the wettest and most suitable for irrigated agriculture. Urban areas are depicted in gray/red respectively

smaller areas just north of Stepanakert/Khankendi and surrounding Agdam. Most of Agdam was destroyed in 1993 and then abandoned. This town was supposed to be transferred to Azerbaijan as part of the 2020 conflict resolution and might be repopulated in the future. The topographic wetness index (TWI, Fig. 5.2B) shows that most of the wetter areas are located around the gentle slopes in southern 1994 era greater Karabakh/augmented Armenia. These areas correspond with the irrigated parts of the region, and there are many towns in the areas along the rivers with higher TWI. TWI is very low for the PR-2020 region, except for a small area just north of Stepanakert/Khankendi.

In addition to changes in forests and croplands, surface water is another important aspect of the land which is relevant to this conflict and its associated epidemic of malaria. Water shortages and droughts are major sources of concern in Azerbaijan (Palazzo 2020). Several important water reservoirs are located on the recaptured lands, such as the large water reservoir in Mataghis which feeds water to the Sarsang water facility and is currently still controlled by Yerevan-backed separatists. Another reservoir in Mataghis is very important for the irrigation of croplands in the southern part of our study region. Before the 2020 conflict, the irrigation canal from Sarsang that fed these croplands was not providing water to Azerbaijani lowland croplands (Palazzo 2020). Abundant water from the mountainous regions fed large river systems for both Armenia and Azerbaijan.

## 5.4 Cropland Abandonment

One recent geographic study evaluated the effect of the Karabakh conflict on land surface by comparing the areas within conflict zones with other areas that did not see direct conflicts (Baumann et al. 2015). These researchers found that 9% of the croplands were abandoned between 1987 and 2000, and only 17% of those fields were recultivated by 2010. Much higher abandonment rates were found in the areas where the actual fighting took place. Cropland abandonment was common after the collapse of the Soviet Union, even in areas without conflict, and a strong correlation of abandonment with elevation and slope has been shown (Müller et al. 2013).

The 1994 era Karabakh/augmented Armenia also had a good deal of irrigated cropland, with open irrigation canals crossing the landscape. Our remote sensing analysis showed significant amounts of cropland to the west and south of Yerevan along the Araks River (Fig. 5.3A). The lowland

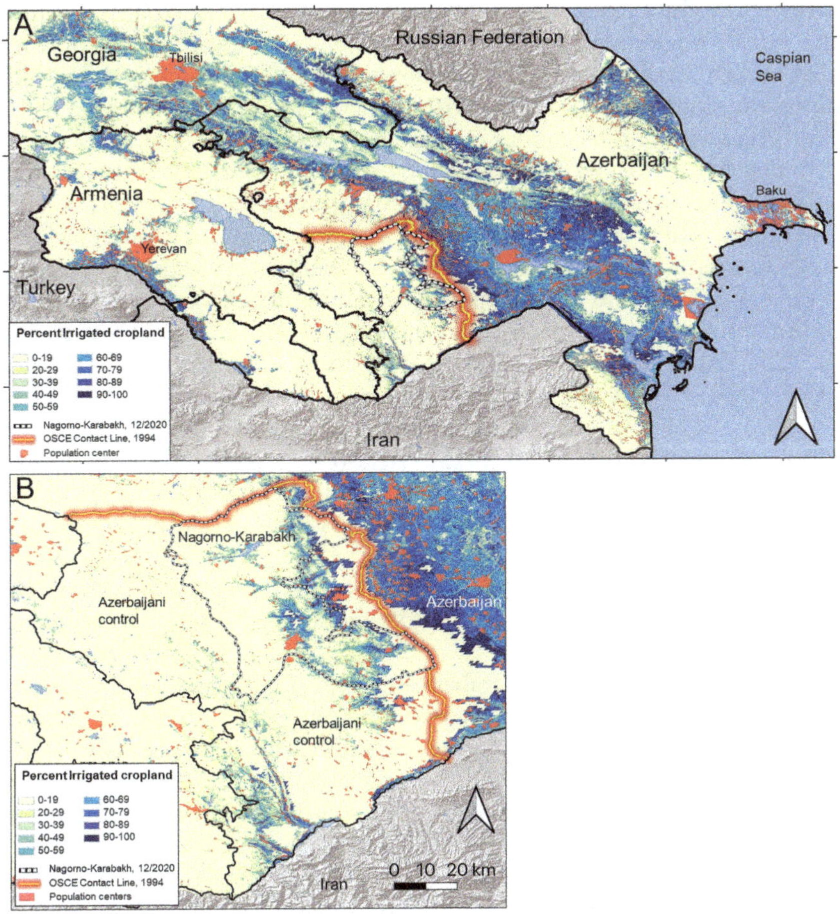


**Fig. 5.3** A (top) and B (bottom) Percent of irrigated cropland by pixel (100x100m, Copernicus Global Land Service dataset) for 2015 in the South Caucasus region (A) and Nagorno-Karabakh region (B). A high percentage of irrigated cropland was found to the west and south of Yerevan, throughout the Kura and Araks River valleys in Azerbaijan and central portions of NGK. The boundaries established in 1994 and at the end of the conflict in the fall of 2020 are shown. Cities and towns are highlighted in red to indicate areas of settlement

areas of the Kura River valley in western and southern Azerbaijan, including border regions with Iran, also indicate a high percent of croplands (Fig. 5.3B). Other areas with croplands in and around central NK and along the south western border with Armenia showed areas of cropland.

To understand the changes in cropland, we used two land cover datasets. The first is the v3.0.1 Copernicus land cover data (Buchhorn et al. 2020), which is available for the years 2015 through 2019 at 100m spatial resolution. This dataset is available at the global scale and provides data both in discrete classes and as continuous field layers with proportional estimates of the land cover types. The data is based on the PROBA-V 100m time series and using high-quality land cover training sites and ancillary datasets has been classified with an accuracy of 80% (Buchhorn et al. 2020). We use the land cover classification where each grid cell is assigned a land cover class to determine the changes in the percentage of croplands between 2015 and 2019. We also use the proportional data to understand in which regions we find more than 10% cropland loss. The second dataset is a regional land cover classification generated for the Caucasus at 30m spatial resolution for the years 1987, 1995, 2000, 2005, 2010 and 2015 (Buchner et al. 2020). Overall accuracy was a little over 80% for this dataset as well, with slightly higher user accuracies for forests than for croplands.

Most of the augmented Karabakh region is either herbaceous vegetation or forested (Fig. 5.4), with croplands confined to the far eastern and southern parts of the region. The reduced Nagorno-Karabakh region negotiated in the 2020 conflict resolution is predominantly forested, with croplands just north of Stepanakert/Khankendi and in the far southeastern part of the region.

There is one year of overlap (2015) between these two land cover datasets. To identify cropland changes in the region, we first compared the cropland percentages by rayon for the two different datasets in the year 2015 (Fig. 5.5).

We found a 5.7% relative loss of cropland area in the entire region of 1994 era greater Karabakh/augmented Armenia between 1987 and 2015 (32.1% to 30.3%), with a 19% relative loss of cropland area in the post-reconfiguration in 2020 (PR-2020) region (29.2% to 23.7%) and just 1.2% in the area that was recaptured by Azerbaijan. This percentage includes croplands that are classified as mixed, meaning that they are classified as cropland in some years and not in other years, without showing consistent gain or loss. Only 2.6% and 2.3% of the area for 1994 era greater

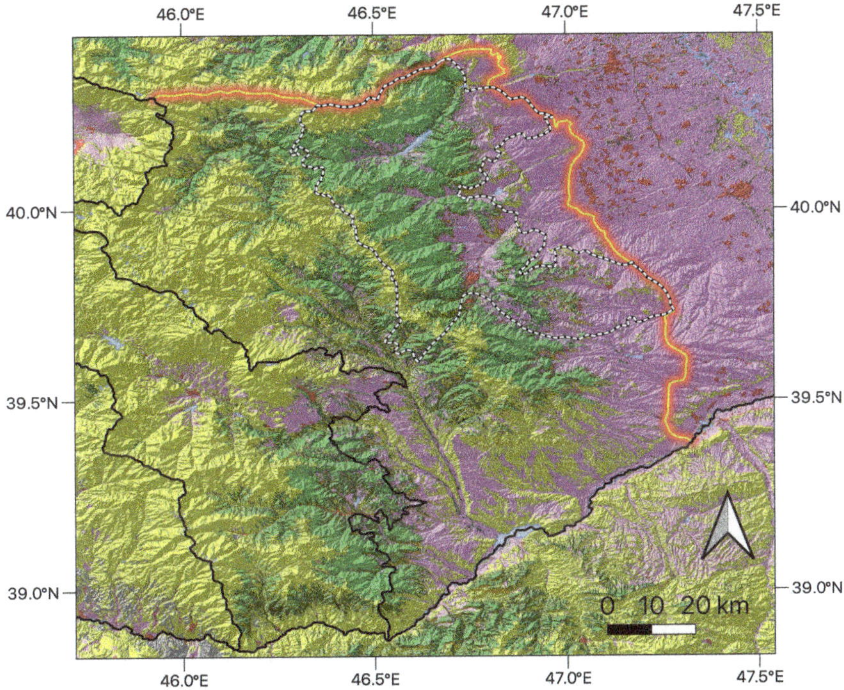


**Fig. 5.4** 2019 Copernicus land cover data at 100m spatial resolution. Green is closed forest, pink is croplands, red is urban and yellow is herbaceous vegetation. The underlying hill shade is based on the SRTM DEM data. Note the very low number of urban areas along the line of contact in Artsakh, compared with the relatively dense number of towns across the line of contact in Azerbaijan. This map shows a substantial amount of cropland in the area between Nagorno-Karabakh and the line of contact. High resolution imagery reveals a mixed story in this region

Karabakh/augmented Armenia and PR-2020, respectively, was classified as cropland the entire time, with 2.7% of the area captured by Azerbaijan in 2020 cropped the entire time. Most of the change occurred in the eastern part of 1994 era greater Karabakh/augmented Armenia (Fig. 5.6A and B), which also has the most cropland (Fig. 5.4). The PR-2020 area has much smaller amounts of cropland than the area recaptured by Azerbaijan in 2020.

The largest cropland relative loss (47%) occurred in Tartar rayon, in the northeastern part of 1994 era greater Karabakh/augmented Armenia. But

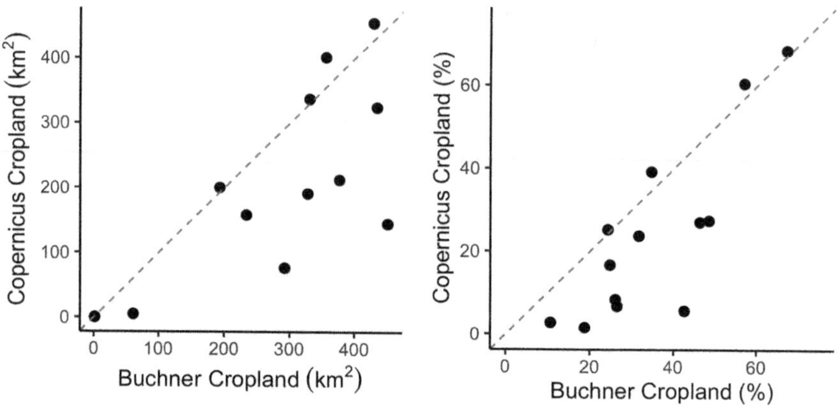


**Fig. 5.5** Cropland area (left, in km²) and cropland percentage (right %) of 13 rayons that make up 1994 era greater Karabakh/augmented Armenia. There is a significant relation between the two cropland area datasets ($p<0.01$) with an $R^2_{adj}$ of 0.5537, although there is more cropland visible in the Buchner dataset than in the Copernicus dataset

several other rayons saw losses of more than 10%. Jabrayil and Fuzuli rayons saw a slight increase in croplands (5.6% and 10.9%), respectively. The Copernicus data reveals a similar pattern in the short period between 2015 and 2019, with the largest decline in percent cropland in Tartar rayon (11.5%) and Agdam rayon (10.6%), surrounding the ghost town of Agdam. Three rayons saw significant increases in croplands: Shusha (43.8%), Kalbajar (28.6%) and Zangilan rayon (14.4%). This dataset shows virtually no change in cropland class, for example from cropland to another land cover class, but 31% of the PR-2020 area revealed a loss in cropland proportion that was more than 10%, for example from 85% cropland in a 100m grid cell, to <75% cropland. The area recaptured by Azerbaijan in 2020 revealed a change greater than 10% in 34% of the region.

The PR-2020 region lost 16.6% of its croplands between 1987 and 1995 as a result of the conflict. The area recently recaptured by Azerbaijan lost 5.9% of its cropland, but much of this was regained in later years. The croplands lost by 1995 had the highest elevation and by far the highest slopes of all the cropland areas lost for both the PR-2020 region and the area recaptured by Azerbaijan. All croplands had higher elevations and steeper slopes in the PR-2020 region than elsewhere in augmented Armenia (Fig. 5.7).

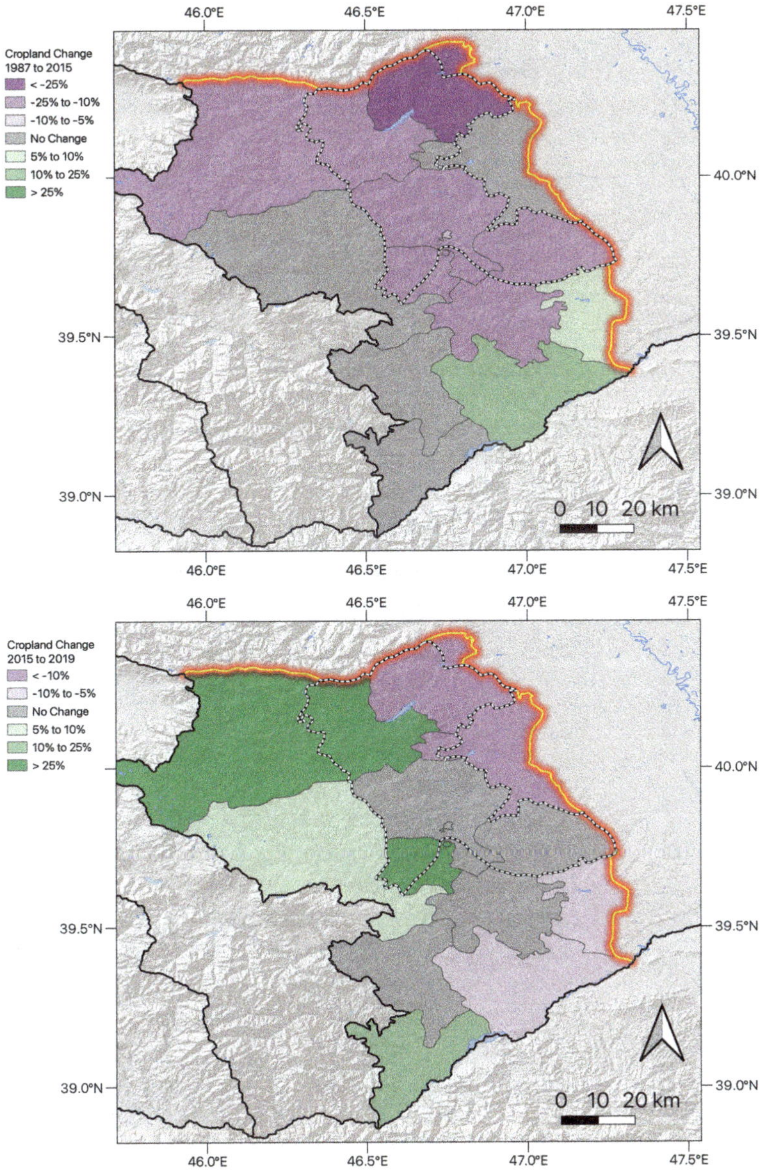


**Fig. 5.6** A (top) and B (bottom): Cropland change between 1987 and 2015 (Figure A top, Buchner et al. 2020), and cropland change between 2015 and 2019 (Figure B bottom, Copernicus)

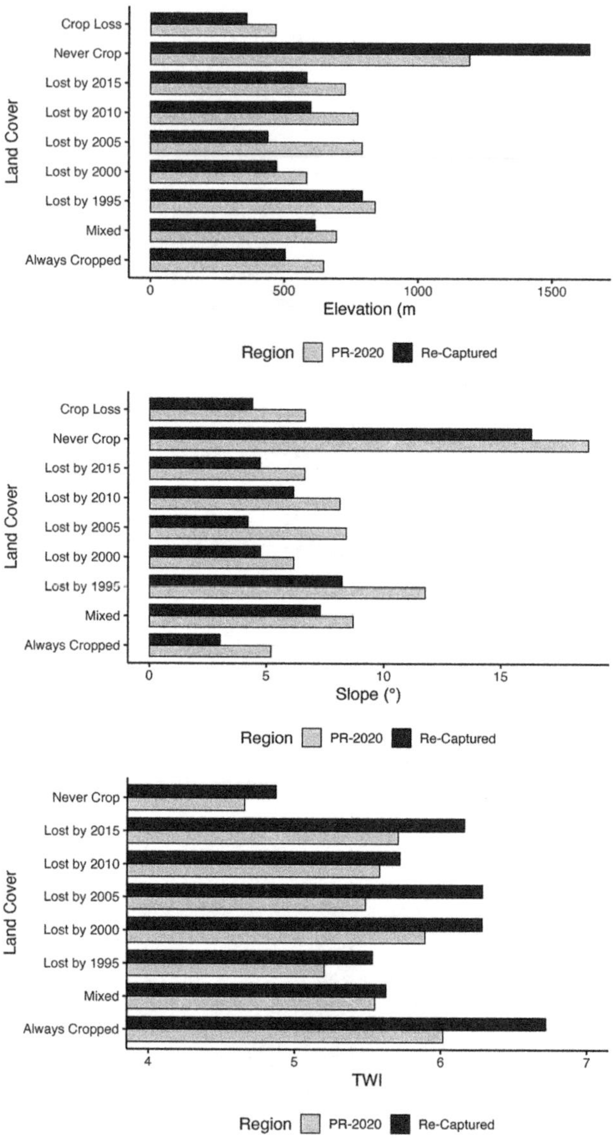


**Fig. 5.7** A (top), B (middle) and C (bottom): Median elevation and slope for the remaining area of post-reconfiguration Nagorno-Karabakh (PR-2020) and the area recaptured by Azerbaijan in the 2020 conflict. Elevation for the areas that are never

The topographic wetness index is also higher for all cropland types in the area recaptured than in PR-2020. The areas that are always cultivated have the highest median TWI, while the areas that are never cultivated have the lowest TWI. Areas abandoned by 1995 had much lower TWI for both regions than areas abandoned at later times (Fig. 5.7A, B and C). Croplands are located on less suitable lands in the PR-2020 region than in the recaptured areas. Close-up imagery shines a light onto the different cropland regions along the line of conflict, for example close to Agdam (Fig. 5.8).

## 5.5 Forest Disturbance

Developed by NASA, the earth-orbiting satellite called Landsat 5 was launched in 1984. We currently have 38 years of global 30m multi-spectral data recorded by four different satellites: Landsat 5, Landsat 7, Landsat 8 and Landsat 9. These satellites record data at a variety of different spectral resolutions and are capable of recording data outside of the regular blue, green and red light that we as humans observe, making them particularly useful for analysis of vegetation changes.

To calculate the forest disturbance index for all years between 2000 and 2020, we select all available images with less than 20% cloud cover between June and August for every year. We then calculate the summer mean for all available images in each year. Next, we process that data into a disturbance index (de Beurs et al. 2016; Healey et al. 2005). We first calculate the Brightness, Greenness and Wetness Tasseled Cap indices (Crist 1985). These indices are linear transformations of the original reflectance data to form indices that are more straightforward to link to the land surface. Next, we standardize these indices against forested areas with at least 80%

**Fig. 5.7** (continued) cropped is higher in the recaptured area, while the elevation for all the cropped areas is higher in PR-2020 (top). The slope of all areas is also greater for the PR-2020 region, indicating a rougher terrain in general (middle). Crop loss represents the area where there was at least 10% cropland loss between 2015 and 2019 according to the Copernicus land cover data (middle). While the slope of the area lost in these last few years is virtually identical to the slope of the area lost by 2015, the elevation is lower, indicating a loss of area from 2015–2019 that is better suitable for croplands. The topographic wetness index (TWI) is always higher for the recently recaptured area, once more indicating better cropland suitability for that region than for PR-2020 (bottom)

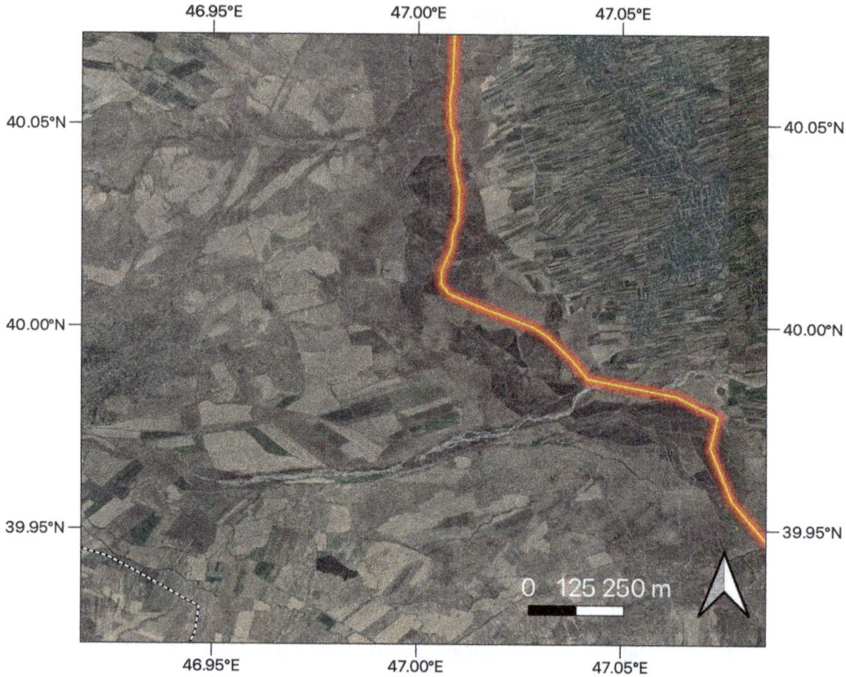


**Fig. 5.8** Croplands along the line of contact between greater Karabakh/augmented Armenia and Azerbaijan. Burned fields are visible along the line of contact. The fields in Azerbaijan are highly fragmented, which happened after the collapse of the Soviet Union. Despite the abandonment of the town of Agdam in the west of the image, some cultivated croplands are still visible in this region

tree cover and no change between 2000 and 2019, using the Hansen Global Forest Change data (Hansen et al. 2013). We also standardize by rayon and aspect, for example, to ensure that north facing slopes are only compared to other north facing slopes. For the aspect standardization we look at north facing, south facing and flat areas (slope <6°). Finally, the disturbance index is calculated as follows:

$$DI = Brightness - (Greenness + Wetness)$$

This index can capture forest disturbance because disturbed forests typically are brighter, less green and less wet than healthy forests.

We compared these forest disturbance data from 2000–2020 with a regional land cover classification developed for the Caucasus (Buchner et al. 2020), which also uses Landsat data, but classifies the data in distinct land cover classes for the years 1987, 1995, 2000, 2005, 2010 and 2015. As a result of the energy embargo, some forested areas were cut after the 1993 conflict to provide a heating source. We evaluated forest loss with two different datasets. First, we compare the total forest percentages by rayon for the overlapping years: 2000, 2005, 2010 and 2015. It is important to realize that these forest cover/disturbance datasets are not generated equally. The Buchner data provides a forest/non-forest classification, while the disturbance index data only incorporates pixels that are at least 80% forest according to the Hansen global forest data and then investigates disturbance of those forests. Next, we evaluate the forest loss with the Buchner data which covers the years 1987, 2000, 2005, 2010 and 2015, and we evaluate forest disturbance data for the years 2000–2020.

A comparison of the undisturbed forests and the areas classified as forest by Buchner et al. (2020; Fig. 5.9) reveals generally strong agreement between the two datasets for all years (Table 5.1).

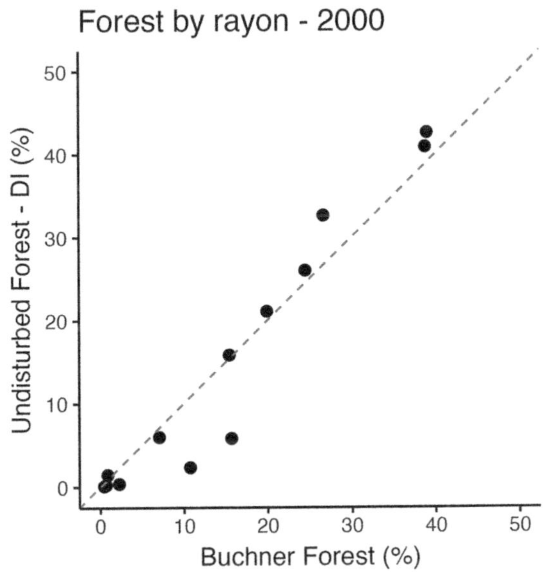


**Fig. 5.9** Percentage of undisturbed forest and the percentage of forest from Buchner et al. (2020) by rayon in 1994 era greater Karabakh/augmented Armenia. The red line provides the 1:1 line. There is a significant relationship between these variables with a slope of 1.13, and an intercept of −2.5% ($R^2_{adj}$ = 0.933)

**Table 5.1** Regression between the percent undisturbed forest according to the disturbance data (DI) and the Buchner forest data (BF)

| *Year* | *Regression equation* | $R^2_{adj}$ | *RSE* |
|---|---|---|---|
| 2000 | *DI* = -2.5%+1.13 *BF* | 0.933 | 4.1 |
| 2005 | *DI* = -2.4%+1.14 *BF* | 0.932 | 4.2 |
| 2010 | *DI* = -2.8%+1.16 *BF* | 0.936 | 4.1 |
| 2015 | *DI* = -4.0%+1.16 *BF* | 0.937 | 4.0 |

The regression relations are very stable, with similar $R^2_{adj}$ and Residual Standard Error (RSE) for each year

If we compare the forest area lost (e.g. forest is classified as another class) and the area disturbed over time, it is clear that while the area lost is small (<30km$^2$ in total, Fig. 5.10A, top), there are many more forests that are disturbed (~200km$^2$, Fig. 5.10B, bottom). We see a strong decline in deforestation after the initial shock in the 1990s and early 2000s, with the total area of deforestation declining from less than 30km$^2$ per year, to less than 10km$^2$ per year by 2010. There is a slight increase in deforestation in 2015.

The amount of deforestation in the area recaptured by Azerbaijan in 2020 is much greater than the amount of deforestation in the remaining area of Nagorno-Karabakh (PR-2020). On the other hand, Fig. 5.11 reveals relatively stable amounts of forest disturbance, with approximately the same area of forests disturbed in PR-2020 as in the recaptured area. It is interesting to note that while the area of clear-cut forests may be relatively small in PR-2020, there is still a lot of forest disturbance. In addition, the latter data reveals a steep increase in forest disturbance in the area recaptured by Azerbaijan. This 2020 disturbance was recorded with data from June–August 2020, before the actual 2020 conflict began.

The elevation of the forested areas is slightly higher than the elevation of the regions that are not forested (Fig. 5.11A, top). Forests at lower elevations were cut first (1995), with forests at higher elevations cut later, although this trend was stronger for the recaptured area than for PR-2020. The slope of the forested areas is greater in both regions than the slope of areas with other land cover types. Both regions reveal that the slope of the areas with forest loss increases steadily, with the lowest slopes for the areas that are lost by 1995, and the highest slopes for areas lost by 2015 (Fig. 5.11B, bottom). In most cases, the slope of the forests that are lost in PR-2020 is slightly higher than the slope of the forests lost in the recaptured area.

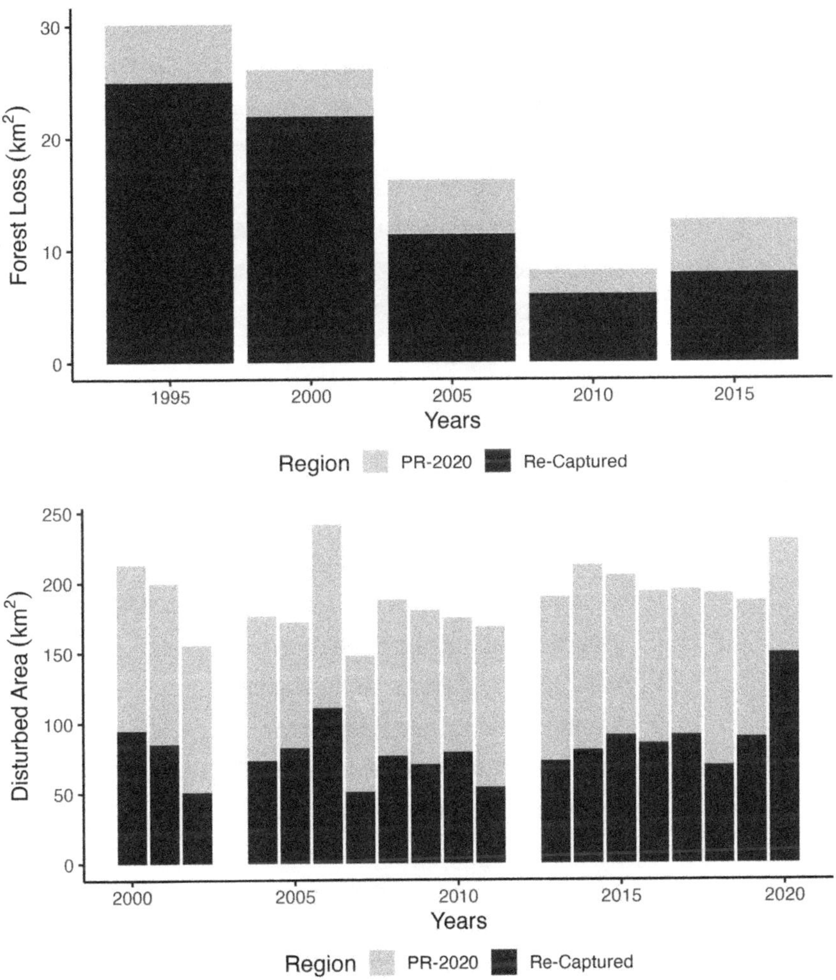


**Fig. 5.10** A (top) and B (bottom): Buchner et al. (2020) forest loss in post 2020 reconfiguration (PR-2020) and in the area recaptured by Azerbaijan (top). Note how the amount of forest loss decreases over time. With the largest area of loss from 1987 to 1995 and the second largest area of loss from 1995 to 2000. Forest disturbance between 2000 and 2020 (bottom). Disturbance and forest loss are not the same, disturbance of a forest is possible even if the forest itself is not lost. Note the large amount of disturbance in 2020

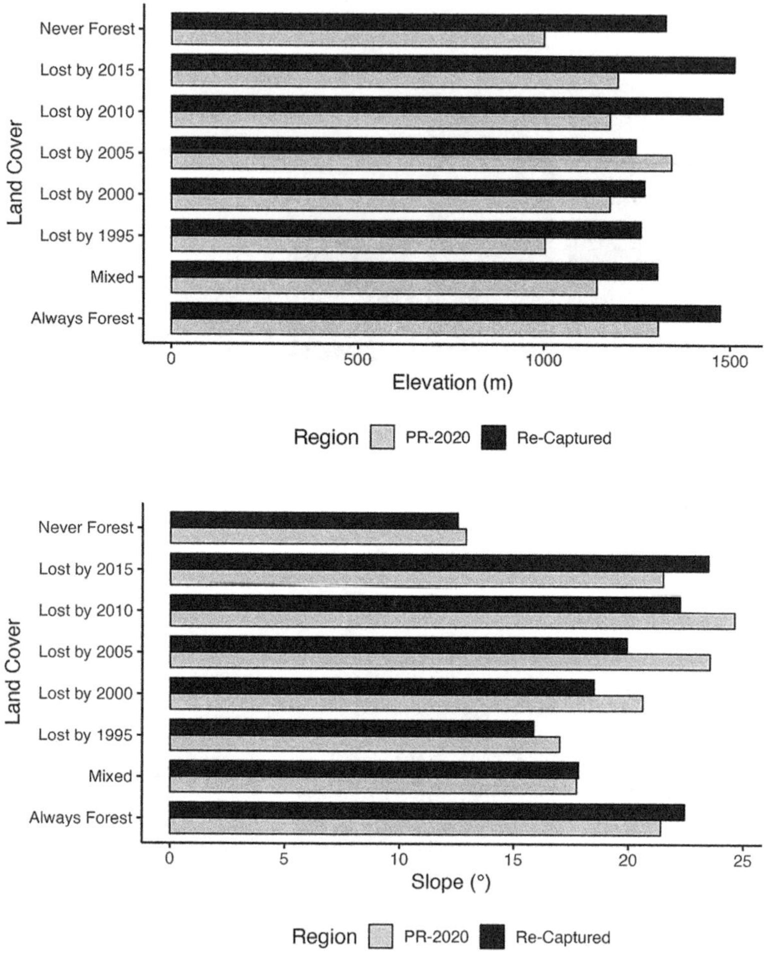


**Fig. 5.11** A (top) and B (bottom): Forest loss data from Buchner et al. (2020) compared with average elevation (top) and slope (bottom)

We used the disturbance index data between 2000 and 2020 to determine how long areas were disturbed and found that 69% of the forests are never disturbed. On the flip side, 3% of the forests are disturbed more than 16 years, with 0.65% of those pixels being disturbed the entire time period. This might indicate that these forests were misclassified at the beginning

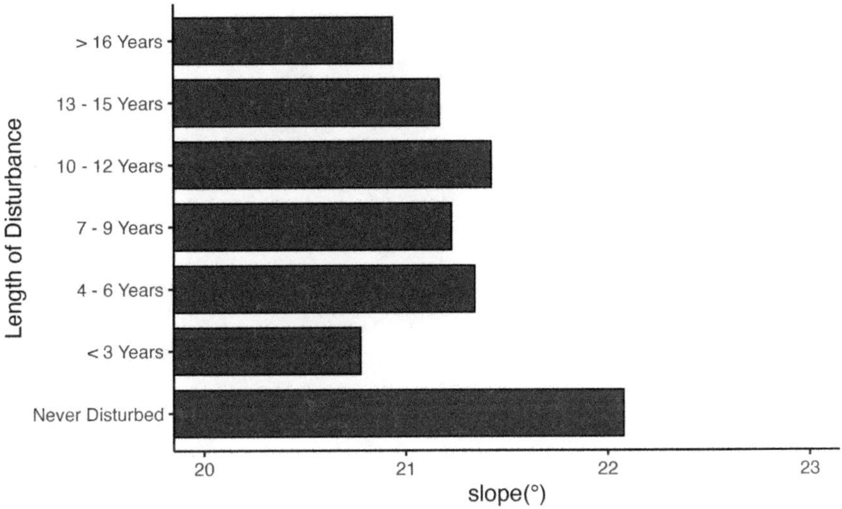


**Fig. 5.12** Slope of the disturbed forests by length of disturbance. The areas that were never disturbed and are continuously classified as forests have the greatest slopes. Gentler slopes are found for areas with less than three years' disturbance. Areas with more than 16 years of disturbance are most likely misclassified areas that were never forests to begin with (<3% of the forests)

of the study period and in fact were never forest. Just below 12% of the forests were disturbed only one year in the full study period, and many of the pixels that were disturbed in 2020 fall in this category. About 4% of the forests were disturbed between two and six years, indicating either disturbance followed by recovery or a disturbance later in the study period. Figure 5.12 provides the slope of the forests by disturbance length. Those areas that were never disturbed had the steepest slopes, while areas that were briefly disturbed had the gentlest slopes. Figure 5.13 illustrates the extent of forest disturbance before and after the resurgence of armed conflict in 2020, and the widespread forest fires that occurred in the areas recaptured by Azerbaijan.

An overview of the socio-economic and environmental impacts of the areas affected by the 2020 conflict is currently available through ACAPS (ACAPS 2020). This report also discusses the increase in fires in 2020 and the subsequent deterioration of air quality but does not investigate the ongoing changes in land cover in the region (ACAPS 2020). The fighting

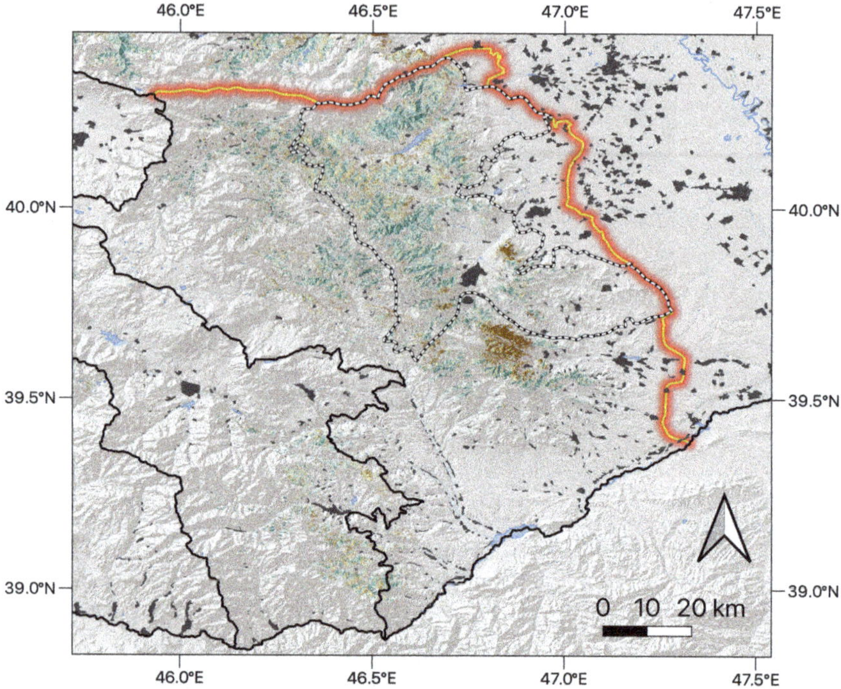


**Fig. 5.13** Forest disturbance (brown) observed in the summer of 2020, before the latest conflict occurred. Large forest disturbances can be seen just south of Shusha in the area that was later captured by Azerbaijan and was a hotspot for 2020 fires (ACAPS 2020). There is also a patch of disturbance northeast of Stepanakert/Khankendi. Urban centers are plotted in dark gray

and political instability during October and November 2020 also appears to have led to an 8- and 30-fold increase in the number of cases of SARS-CoV-2 infections in both Armenia and Azerbaijan, respectively, compared to before the conflict (Kazaryan et al. 2020). Case numbers in Nagorno-Karabakh are hard to determine, but news outlets reported dramatic increases in Stepanakert and Shusha during the war as residents were forced to live in close quarters and underground shelters (CTV News 2020; AP News 2020). After 30 years, conflict continues and residents are still susceptible to political, economic, and social instability, as well as new disease outbreaks.

The process of rebordering that began with the Karabakh conflict is still unresolved. Armenia and Azerbaijan both maintain "rival topographies" with place names, landmarks and administrative boundaries rendered differently in Armenian and Azerbaijani maps (Broers 2021: xiii). This cartographic uncertainty even extends to the digital realm. In December 2021 the Government of Azerbaijan formally petitioned Google maps to remove Armenian place names from the Karabakh region (Asbarez 2021). Several mapping apps continue to show different place names depending on the viewer's location. As one recent report described,

> Yandex Maps shows a road neatly aligned to the international border, while Google puts long stretches squarely in Azerbaijani territory. The community-derived Open Street Map also shows the road crossing into Azerbaijan but not quite in the same way that Google does, placing a bit more of the curving road north of Shurnukh on the Azerbaijani side. None of these platforms have access to special information on the border demarcation process, but all of them do a good job at creating the illusion of geographic authority. (McGlynn 2021)

This has created problems for travelers who rely on centralized internet sources such as GoogleMaps for navigating the region only to discover that the maps can be quite different depending on where they are accessed (McGlynn 2021). In December 2021 the Government of Azerbaijan formally requested Google to remove Armenian place names from Karabakh maps (Asbarez.com 2021). All this geopolitical and cartographic uncertainty has made Karabakh tricky to navigate and much of the region remains underpopulated.

## References

ACAPS. 2020. Azerbaijan: Pre-existing Situation and Impact of the 2020 Nagorno Karabakh Conflict. December 2020. https://www.acaps.org/sites/acaps/files/products/files/20201221_acaps_secondary_data_review_azerbaijan_nagorno-karabakh_conflict.pdf. Accessed March 2021.

AP (Associated Press) News. 2020. Coronavirus Spreads in Nagorno-Karabakh amid Heavy Fighting. October 21. https://apnews.com/article/virus-outbreak-pandemics-azerbaijanarmenia-europe-14f519a45ce899c2c7a52cba7c876850. Accessed March 2020.

Asbarez. 2021. Baku Urges Google Maps to Remove Armenian Names from Karabakh Map. https://asbarez.com/baku-urges-google-maps-to-remove-armenian-namesfrom-karabakh-map/. Accessed 6 September 2022.

Baumann, Matthias, Volker Radeloff, Vahagn Avedian, and Tobias Kuemmerle. 2015. Land Use Change in the Caucasus During and After the Nagorno-Karabakh Conflict. *Regional Environmental Change* 15 (8): 1703–1716.

Broers, Laurence. 2021. *Armenia and Azerbaijan: Anatomy of a Rivalry.* Edinburgh: Edinburgh University Press.

Buchhorn, Marcel, Myroslava Lesiv, Nandin-Erdene Tsendbazar, Martin Herold, Luc Bertels, and Bruno Smets. 2020. Copernicus Global Land Cover Layers—Collection 2. *Remote Sensing* 12 (6): 1044. https://doi.org/10.3390/rs12061044.

Buchner, Johanna, He Yin, David Frantz, Tobias Kuemmerle, Elshad Askerov, Tamar Bakuradze, Benjamin Bleyhl, Nodar Elizbarashvili, Anna Komarova, Katarzyna E. Lewińska, Afag Rizayeva, Hovik Sayadyan, Bin Tank, Garegin Tepanosyan, Nugzar Zazanashvilie, and Volker C. Radeloff. 2020. Land-Cover Change in the Caucasus Mountains since 1987 Based on the Topographic Correction of Multi-temporal Landsat Composites. *Remote Sensing of Environment* 248: 111967.

Cookman, Liz. 2020. For Armenians Fleeing Nagorno-Karabakh, 'Losing It Is Everything.' Foreign Policy. November 20 https://foreignpolicy.com/2020/11/20/armenians-fleeingnagorno-karabakh-bitter-peace/. Accessed 29 October 2022.

Crisis Group. 2022a. Warding Off Renewed War in Nagorno-Karabakh. https://www.crisisgroup.org/europe-central-asia/caucasus/nagorno-karabakh-conflict/warding-renewed-war-nagorno-karabakh. Accessed 22 September 2022.

———. 2022b. The Nagorno-Karabakh Conflict: A Visual Explainer. https://www.crisisgroup.org/content/nagorno-karabakh-conflict-visual-explainer. Accessed 29 October 2022.

———. 2022c. Upholding the Ceasefire between Azerbaijan and Armenia. September 28. https://www.crisisgroup.org/europe-central-asia/caucasus/armenia-azerbaijannagorno-karabakh-conflict/upholding-ceasefire. Accessed 29 October 2022.

Crist, Eric P. 1985. A TM Tasseled Cap Equivalent Transformation for Reflectance Factor Data. *Remote Sens. Environ.* 17: 301–306.

CTV News. 2020. Coronavirus Thrives in Karabakh's Bomb Shelters. October 24. https://www.ctvnews.ca/health/coronavirus/coronavirus-thrives-in-karabakh-s-bomb-shelters-1.5159270. Accessed March 2020.

de Beurs, Kirsten, Braden C. Owsley, and Jason P. Julian. 2016. Disturbance Analyses of Forests and Grasslands with MODIS and Landsat in New Zealand. *International Journal of Applied Earth Observation and Geoinformation.* https://doi.org/10.1016/j.jag.2015.10.009.

de Waal, Thomas. 2017. The Threat of a Karabakh Conflict in 2017. Carnegie Europe. https://carnegieeurope.eu/strategiceurope/67774. Accessed 11 September 2022.

———. 2021. Unfinished Business in the Armenia-Azerbaijan Conflict. Carnegie Europe. https://carnegieeurope.eu/2021/02/11/unfinished-business-in-armeniaazerbaijan-conflict-pub-83844. Accessed 29 October 2022.

Glantz, Mary. 2022. *Amid Ukraine War, Armenia and Azerbaijan Fighting Risks Broader Conflict*. United States Institute for Peace. September 15. https://www.usip.org/publications/2022/09/amid-ukraine-war-armenia-and-azerbaijan-fighting-risks-broaderconflict. Accessed 29 October 2022.

Global Conflict Tracker. 2022. Nagorno-Karabakh Conflict. https://www.cfr.org/global-conflict-tracker/conflict/nagorno-karabakh-conflict. Accessed 29 October 2022.

Hansen, Matthew C., Peter V. Potapov, Rebecca Moore, Matthew Hancher, Svetlana A. Turubanova, Alexandra Tyukavina, David Thau, Stephen V. Stehman, Scott J. Goetz, Thomas R. Loveland, Anil Kommareddy, Alexey Egorov, Louise Chini, Christopher O. Justice, and John R.G. Townshend. 2013. High-Resolution Global Maps of 21st-Century Forest Cover Change. *Science* 342 (6160): 850–853.

Healey, Sean P., Warren B. Cohen, Yang Zhiqiang, and Olga N. Krankinab. 2005. Comparison of Tasseled Cap-based Landsat Data Structures for Use in Forest Disturbance Detection. *Remote Sensing of Environment* 97: 301–310.

Isayev, Heydar. 2022. Azerbaijan Announces Plans to Erase Armenian Traces from Churches. *Eurasianet*. https://eurasianet.org/azerbaijan-announces-plans-to-erase-armeniantraces-from-churches. Accessed 29 October 2022.

Kazaryan, Airazat M., Bjørn Edwin, Ara Darzi, Gevorg N. Tamamyan, Mushegh A. Sahakyan, Davit L. Aghayan, Åsmund A. Fretland, Sheraz Yaqub, Brice Gayet, and Doctors Against The War collaborators. 2020. War in the Time of COVID-19: Humanitarian Catastrophe in Nagorno-Karabakh and Armenia. *The Lancet Global Health* 9 (3): 243–244.

Kucera, Joshua. 2020. Armenians Flee Fighting in Karabakh. Eurasianet. November 4. https://eurasianet.org/armenians-flee-fighting-in-karabakh. Accessed 29 October 2022.

Maghakyan, Simon. 2022. Cultural Desecration is Racial Discrimination. Foreign Policy. https://foreignpolicy.com/2022/01/13/armenia-azerbaijan-nagorno-karabakh-culturaldesecration-is-racial-discrimination/. Accessed 29 October 2022.

McGlynn, Evangeline. 2021. On the Armenia-Azerbaijan Border, the Map is Not the Territory. *Eurasianet*. March 15. https://eurasianet.org/perspectives-on-the-armenia-azerbaijanborder-the-map-is-not-the-territory. Accessed 6 September 2022.

Müller, Daniel, Pedro J. Leitão, and Thomas Sikorc. 2013. Comparing the Determinants of Cropland Abandonment in Albania and Romania Using Boosted Regression Trees. *Agricultural Systems* 117: 66–77.

Nutt, David. 2022. Report Shows Near Total Erasure of Armenian Heritage Sites. https://news.cornell.edu/stories/2022/09/report-shows-near-total-erasure-armenian-heritagesites. Accessed 29 October 2022.

Palazzo, Claudia. 2020. *The Water Factor in the Karabakh Conflict*. The Jamestown Foundation Commentary. https://jamestown.org/the-water-factor-in-the-karabakh-conflict. Accessed 23 September 2022.

Sestanovich, Stephen. 2020. Has Russia Really Ended the War between Armenia and Azerbaijan? Council on Foreign Relations. https://www.cfr.org/in-brief/has-russia-endedwar-between-armenia-and-azerbaijan. Accessed 29 October 2022.

Spencer, John, and Harshen Ghoorhoo. 2021. *The Battle of Shusha City and the Missed Lessons of the 2020 Nagorno-Karabakh War*. Modern War Institute. https://mwi.usma.edu/the-battle-of-shusha-city-and-the-missed-lessons-of-the-2020-nagorno-karabakhwar//. Accessed 29 October 2022.

CHAPTER 6

# Conclusions

**Abstract** This chapter summarizes the key lessons learned from this work. We conclude that Mary Kaldor's concept of "New Wars" is useful for understanding the unique environmental and human impacts of contemporary armed conflicts. Combining qualitative historical research with remote sensing data provides insights into these dynamics. Specifically our research leads us to conclude that the Karabakh conflict and the Soviet collapse led to a prolonged period of violence and territorial uncertainty for the Karabakh region. Forced migration left thousands of Armenians and Azeris crowded in makeshift camps and improvised housing at a time when public health prevention measures were largely absent. The war itself generated "ecological insults" to the land creating conditions favorable for mosquito habitat. We conclude by presenting Valery Tishkov's concept of "demodernization" and argue that New Wars have the potential to rapidly shift mortality from non-infectious to infectious and vector borne diseases in societies that have achieved a "modern" health profile.

**Keywords** Demodernization • Environmental insults • Territorial uncertainty • Refugee crises

Our primary goal in this collaborative work has been to combine qualitative historical and social science research with geospatial analysis to better understand the relationship between armed conflict, environmental



K. Hirschfeld et al., *New Wars and Old Plagues*,
https://doi.org/10.1007/978-3-031-31143-7_6

change and population health crises in the Caucasus. As Mary Kaldor has described, New Wars like the Karabakh conflict are different from the nation-state warfare that defined the twentieth century (2012). New War armies are more likely to begin as informal militias, and violence against civilians is common.

A number of scholars in public health and global health have identified New War conflicts and "resource wars" as contributing to disease outbreaks, but the mechanisms driving these health transitions have not been fully established (Bausch and Schwarz 2014; Hotez 2020; Klare et al. 2011). Our extended case study explores the Karabakh conflict and its associated health crises through an expanded temporal and spatial lens that better contextualizes the population health crises that accompanied this conflict.

Our historical analysis, for instance, reveals that *P. vivax* was well established in northern latitudes prior to the Soviet eradication campaign. This suggests the malaria epidemic in the 1990s should not be viewed as an anomalous outbreak of a tropical disease in a temperate zone, but as the return of an ancestral pathogen with a long history of success in the region. Our geospatial analysis provides insight into the ways warfare changed the natural environment in the Caucasus to facilitate sustained transmission of malaria and other preventable infectious diseases.

One key process that contributed to the health crisis that emerged during the Karabakh conflict in the 1990s was the reconfiguration of political boundaries following the collapse of the USSR. These processes are not well theorized in political science or international relations (Mandic 2021). Both fields remain influenced by twentieth-century beliefs about the permanency of Westphalian states, and there is less consensus about the inverse processes of state fragmentation, collapse or territorial reconfiguration (Fituni 1995; Mandic 2021; Rich 1999; Zartman 1995). But many New War conflicts are driven by ethnic or other separatists that create "torn states" with uncertain territorial boundaries (Mandic 2021). In his detailed study of the Karabakh conflict, Laurence Broers referred to this process as "rebordering" (2021).

Rebordering signifies the reconfiguration of geopolitical boundaries through the creation of new semi-autonomous mini-statelets (like Karabakh in the early 1990s) as well as the violent incorporation of contested borderlands into existing nation-states.

Our research leads us to expand this concept by dividing it into phases. Rebordering is preceded by "debordering," or the coercive extraction of territory from one nation-state prior to incorporation into another. This work is typically done by violent non-state actors, such as ethnic militias, organized crime groups or warlords who often go on to become political leaders in breakaway regions (Mandic 2021).

Debordering is inherently violent and creates tremendous human vulnerability, including vulnerability to infectious diseases. There are no formal rules of engagement governing warfare between non-state actors. Atrocities, human rights abuses and attacks on infrastructure (including hospitals and health care facilities) are common (Gall and De Waal 1997; Gilman et al. 2015; Trabulsi 2015). Insurgencies are often financed with activities in the informal economy and may include collaborations or transactions with international organized crime groups (Broers 2021; Glenny 2008; Mandic 2021; Zurcher 2007). Warlordism is a common feature of governance in breakaway regions (Bunker 2015; Chan 1999; Mandic 2021; Marten 2012; Rich 1999; Sullivan 2015).

In the early phases of the Karabakh conflict ethnic militias waged internal warfare that resulted in mass killing of civilians and expulsion of minority populations from contested regions. The surrounding nation-state—the USSR—then used violence against militias to try and re-establish control of breakaway territories. In the spring of 1991 the Soviet army launched "Operation Ring," and encircled multiple Armenian villages. Electricity and communications were cut off and Armenians were forcibly removed for the crime of articulating an anti-Soviet national identity (Croissant 1998; de Waal 2013: 116). Atrocities were common, similar to the ones perpetrated by Soviet soldiers during their occupation of Afghanistan in the 1980s (Gall and De Waal 1997). After the Soviet Union collapsed in 1991, Armenia mounted a new offensive and reclaimed a good deal of territory that had been repopulated by Azeri settlers during Operation Ring. Ongoing military successes led to Armenia to claim an additional 7100 square kilometers around Karabakh that had previously been part of Azerbaijan during the Soviet era (Broers 2021: 269). Renewed hostilities in the winter of 2020 led to further revision of the region's cartography and significant territory controlled by Armenia was returned to Azerbaijan as part of a peace deal.

During the early phase of conflict in the late 1980s and early 1990s, disease surveillance and vector control activities were interrupted due to the collapse of the USSR and the devastating 1988 earthquake. Population mobility accelerated due to forced migration of refugees. New groups entered the region, including foreign fighters from malaria prone areas of Afghanistan and Turkey. Once malaria was imported there were few obstacles to sustained transmission due to the collapse of government services and the crowding of vulnerable populations into improvised housing and refugee camps.

Sonia Shah has described how warfare generates "ecological insults" to the landscape that create environmental conditions favorable for mosquito breeding and malaria transmission. Some of these activities include digging trenches, destruction of dams and construction of new roads through uninhabited areas (2010: 86). In the Karabakh conflict, our remote sensing analysis identified multiple environmental insults that very likely contributed to the re-emergence and expansion of malaria in lowland areas surrounding the primary conflict zone. There were high rates of forest disturbance, for instance, as remote villages were cut off from fuel supplies and rural households harvested timber to heat their homes. Criminal groups allegedly took advantage of weak or absent governance to engage in illegal logging or natural resource extraction that further destabilized the natural environment (Conflict and Environment Observatory 2021; UNECE 2019).

Other environmental insults in the Caucasus included high rates of cropland abandonment and changes in surface water resulting from clogged irrigation canals. Abandoned farmland, especially when fed by open irrigation canals like in the Caucasus, provides an ideal habitat for anopheles mosquitos. This is one reason Soviet malaria control efforts in the 1920s and 1930s required an extensive workforce to monitor rural areas and waterways for signs of Anopheles mosquito activity (Johnson 1988). Despite this massive investment in public health and engineering work malaria remained endemic in the USSR until the widespread use of DDT in the 1950s.

A brief survey of other post-Cold War conflicts in the Caucasus reveals similar patterns of violent rebordering accompanied by forced migration and population health crises (Guha-Sapir and van Panhuis 2002; Levy and Sidel 2016; WHO 2019). Georgia suffered three civil wars in the 1990s that led to over 250,000 people being displaced from the Abkhazia region due to ethnic violence (Zurcher 2007). During that time multiple armed groups occupied different sections of the country, engaged in informal taxation and "combined 'patriotic' with purely profit seeking motivations" (Zurcher 2007: 146).

The conflict in Georgia also triggered outbreaks of malaria, with hundreds of cases recorded between the early 1990s and 2000s (Kandelaki et al. 2012). Reduced health budgets, collapse of infrastructure and interruption of malaria prevention measures were all identified as contributing factors in these outbreaks (Sabatinelli 2002). The majority of cases in Georgia were reported in the eastern portions of the country along the borders with Azerbaijan and Armenia. The consequences of the conflict in these countries, including large-scale population migrations likely exacerbated the expansion of malaria in Georgia.

Civil war also broke out in Tajikistan following the collapse of the Soviet Union, with malaria cases increasing from approximately 400 per year in 1992 to nearly 30,000 in 1998 (Matthys et al. 2008). Many factors have been implicated in the malaria re-emergence in Tajikistan (and other former Soviet Republics), including reduced pesticide spraying, planting of crops such as rice and cotton. The influx of refugees, including nearly 600,000 ethnic Tajiks from malaria prone regions of Afghanistan, also contributed to the expansion of epidemic malaria throughout the region (Kondrashin et al. 2017; Sabatinelli 2002). Malaria control measures were intensified in 1999 but it took nearly ten years of sustained public health work to achieve full elimination (Kondrashin et al. 2017).

In Chechnya, years of irregular conflict and unresolved attempts at rebordering in the 1990s resulted in the complete destruction of urban infrastructure and rapid breakdown of the social order. According to Valery Tishkov, "civilian casualties in the Chechen war have exceeded those of both Russia's army and the insurgents' battalions and guerrillas" (2004: xiii). Approximately 400,000 people—one-third of the population—became displaced by conflict in Chechnya and 35,000 were killed (2004: xiii). Kidnappings and homicides—including indiscriminate killing of foreign aid workers and journalists—were common. Enterprising warlords and other *biznesmen-patrioty* seized control of agricultural areas and engaged in massive deforestation for poppy cultivation (2004: 188). The prolonged conflict in Chechnya reduced industrial production in the region to levels representing only about 5% of prewar production (2004: 188). Schools and health facilities closed and the homicide rate increased 700% (2004: 66). Journalists Carlotta Gall and Thomas de Waal described Chechnya in 1994 as "a Shakespearean kingdom with armed groups roaming the countryside at will… [with] no fixed borders or front lines" (1997: 137).

Valery Tishkov detailed how the conflict in Chechnya created "pre-modern" social conditions due to the rapid exodus of educated professionals from the region (2004). Tishkov observed that the exodus of educated professionals from conflict zones makes "the agenda of modern life" impossible to maintain (2004: 14). The result is a return to a pre-modern social order: kin-based social organization reinforced by ethnic and religious homogeneity. The state's monopoly on violence disappears and clan-based communal violence expands to regulate social and economic life. Populations became desensitized as "accepted limitations on violence are abandoned and society increasingly lapses into anarchy and chaos" (2004: 127). Tishkov describes these institutional changes as combining to create a process he terms "demodernization" (2004: 13).

Our research suggests that New Wars, in addition to demodernizing social institutions, can also generate demodernization of health and mortality patterns. To elaborate, a "modern" mortality profile is one where the majority of deaths in a population are from non-infectious diseases of older age groups like heart disease and cancer (Barrett and Armelagos 2014; Schneider 2014). Modern health indicators are achieved by a combination of public health interventions (such as clean water and sanitation systems) combined with improved nutrition, lower fertility rates and consistent childhood immunizations (Barrett and Armelagos 2014). A "pre-modern" health and mortality pattern, on the other hand, is one with high death rates from acute infectious diseases—especially childhood diseases like measles, diphtheria and typhoid. During the late Soviet period all the Caucasus countries reported relatively modern health and mortality patterns (Cockerham 1999). But multiple New War conflicts in the 1990s led to extensive outbreaks of "pre-modern" diseases—including malaria—in these "modern" societies.

During the twentieth century most public health professionals regarded modernization of health as a one-way process (Barrett and Armelagos 2014; Omran 1971). Once a society has successfully controlled preventable infectious diseases, those successes were assumed to be more or less permanent. These beliefs were formalized in "demographic transition theory," which still appears as a regular feature in some public health textbooks and teaching materials (Barrett and Armelagos 2014; Schneider 2014). While many public health scholars have recognized the growing risks of emerging infectious diseases and new pandemics (Hotez 2020; Shah 2016) there has not yet been a formal revision of mortality transition theory to include reverse transitions that temporarily or permanently return a population to pre-modern health and mortality patterns.

Our research suggests that New War conflicts, especially those with multiple cycles of debordering and rebordering, have this potential. Debordering creates rapid environmental changes from armed conflict and the expansion of "ungoverned spaces," devoid of essential public services. Incomplete rebordering can lead to prolonged depopulation of regions and parallel expansion of crowded refugee settlements and improvised housing in neighboring areas. Ethnic minorities are likely to be expelled from homes and farmsteads, leaving behind abandoned land. If new settlers move into the region, they become vulnerable to retaliatory violence if the conflict reignites or expands. In Karabakh some villages experienced repeated waves of forced migration, violence and resettlement during the most intense years of conflict between 1988–1994. All these trends create conditions of demodernization, with a return to informal kin-based systems of governance and exchange. Demodernization of the social world also sets the stage for demodernization of health and mortality patterns, as the infrastructure of infectious disease control contracts or collapses in contested territories.

Even without sustained conflict re-emerging in the Caucasus, the population impacts of climate change are likely to create similar health crises in vulnerable regions. Rising sea levels and ocean temperatures are increasing extreme weather events around the world (IPCC AR5 2014). Outbreaks of vector-borne diseases, including malaria, dengue and tick-borne diseases, are increasingly common outside of their established twentieth-century risk zones (Smith et al. 2014). Waterborne diseases such as cholera are common in flood-stricken areas with limited infrastructure (Smith et al. 2014: 726). Repeated extreme events in the same location may create prolonged cycles of economic and social instability, including violent resource competition that occasionally flares into a New War. These changes will increase population movements and outbreaks of preventable infectious diseases, including "tropical" diseases like malaria in temperate zones (Hotez 2016, 2020).

The conflict in Karabakh reignited in December 2020 and some of the areas claimed by Armenia in 1994 were returned to Azerbaijan as part of a peace deal brokered by Russia. There is still no formal consensus about the geographic revisions, and low intensity violence continues to erupt in contested areas (Hernandez 2022). The southern Caucasus may not yet be done with rebordering and the possibility of new conflict and associated health and environmental crises remains high.

## References

Barrett, Ron, and George Armelagos. 2014. *An Unnatural History of Emerging Infections*. Oxford: Oxford University Press.

Bausch, Daniel G., and Lara Schwarz. 2014. Outbreak of Ebola Virus Disease in Guinea: Where Ecology Meets Economy. *PLOS Neglected Tropical Diseases* 8 (7) https://www.ncbi.nlm.nih.gov/pmc/articles/PMC4117598/. Accessed 26 September 2022.

Broers, Laurence. 2021. *Armenia and Azerbaijan: Anatomy of a Rivalry*. Edinburgh: Edinburgh University Press.

Bunker, Robert. 2015. Forward: Violent Entrepreneurs and Techno Warlords: All Edge. In *Warlords, Inc., Black Markets, Broken States and the Rise of the Warlord Entrepreneur*, ed. Noah Raford and Andrew Trabulsi, 13–26. Berkeley: North Atlantic Books.

Chan, Stephen. 1999. The Warlord and Global Order. In *Warlords in International Relations*, ed. Paul Rich, 164–172. New York: St. Martin's Press.

Cockerham, William. 1999. *Health and Social Change in Russia and Eastern Europe*. New York: Routledge.

Conflict and Environment Observatory. 2021. Report: Investigating the Environmental Dimensions of the 2020 Nagorno Karabakh Conflict. https://ceobs.org/investigating-theenvironmental-dimensions-of-the-nagorno-karabakh-conflict/. Accessed 2 October 2022.

Croissant, Michael. 1998. *The Armenia-Azerbaijan Conflict: Causes and Implications*. Westport, CT: Praeger.

Fituni, Leonid. 1995. The Collapse of the Socialist State: Angola and the Soviet Union. In *Collapsed States: The Disintegration and Restoration of Legitimate Authority*, ed. William Zartman, 143–156. Boulder: Lynne Reinner.

Gall, Carlotta, and Thomas De Waal. 1997. *Chechnya: A Small Victorious War*. London: Pan Books.

Gilman, Nils, Jesse Goldhammer, and Steven Weber. 2015. Innovation, Deviation and Development: Warlords in Proto-State Division. In *Warlords, Inc.*, ed. Noah Raford and Andrew Trabulsi, 108–135. Berkeley: North Atlantic Books.

Glenny, Misha. 2008. *McMafia: A Journey through the Global Criminal Underworld*. New York: Vintage Books.

Guha-Sapir, Debarati, and Willem G. van Panhuis. 2002. *Armed Conflict and Public Health: A Report on Knowledge and Knowledge Gaps*. World Health

Organization Collaborating Centre for Research on the Epidemiology of Disasters (CRED), Catholic University of Louvain. Brussels: CRED. https://reliefweb.int/report/world/armed-conflict-and-public-health-report-knowledge-and-knowledge-gaps.

Hernandez, Joe. 2022. The Deadly Clashes between Armenia and Azerbaijan, Explained. *National Public Radio*. https://www.npr.org/2022/09/19/1123515328/armenia-azerbaijan-nagorno-karabakh-explained. Accessed 2 October 2022.

Hotez, Peter. 2016. *Blue Marble Health: An Innovative Plan to Fight Diseases of the Poor Amid Wealth*. Baltimore: Johns Hopkins University Press.

———. 2020. NTDs in the 2020: An Epic Struggle of Effective Control Tools Versus the Anthropocene. *PLOS Neglected Tropical Diseases* 14 (9) https://journals.plos.org/plosntds/article?id=10.1371/journal.pntd.0007872. Accessed 26 September 2022.

Johnson, Richard. 1988. *Malaria and Malaria Control in the USSR*, 1917–1941. PhD thesis, Georgetown University Department of History.

Kaldor, Mary. 2012. *Old and New Wars*. Malden, MA: Polity Press.

Kandelaki, George, Maia Butsashvili, Irine Kalandadze, Merab Iosava, Nato Avaliana, and Paata Imnadze. 2012. Elimination of Malaria in Country Georgia. *Acta Tropica* 123 (1): 47–48.

Klare, Michael, Barry Levy, and Victor Sidel. 2011. The Public Health Implications of Resource Wars. *American Journal of Public Health* 101 (9): 1615–1619. https://www.ncbi.nlm.nih.gov/pmc/articles/PMC3154227/. Accessed 26 September 2022.

Kondrashin, Anatoly, Azizullo S. Sharipov, Dilshod S. Kadamov, Saifuddin S. Karimov, Elkhan Gasimov, Alla M. Baranova, Lola F. Morozova, Ekaterina V. Stepanova, Natalia A. Turbabina, Maria S. Maksimova, and Evgeny N. Morozov. 2017. Elimination of *Plasmodium falciparum* Malaria in Tajikistan. *Malaria Journal* 16 (226) https://malariajournal.biomedcentral.com/articles/10.1186/s12936-017-1861-5. Accessed 16 September 2022.

Levy, Barry, and Victor Sidel. 2016. Documenting the Effects of Armed Conflict on Population Health. *Annual Reviews of Public Health* 37: 205–218.

Mandic, Danilo. 2021. *Gangsters and Other Statesmen*. Princeton: Princeton University Press.

Marten, Kimberly. 2012. *Warlords: Strong-Arm Brokers in Weak States*. Ithaca: Cornell University Press.

Matthys, Barbara, Tohir Sherkanov, Saifudin Karimov, Zamonidin Khabirov, Till Mostowlansky, Jürg Utzinger, and Kaspar Wyss. 2008. History of Malaria Control in Tajikistan and Rapid Malaria Appraisal in an Agro-Ecological Setting. *Malaria Journal* 7: 217. https://pubmed.ncbi.nlm.nih.gov/18950536/. Accessed 16 September 2022.

Omran, Abel. 1971. The Epidemiological Transition: A Theory of the Epidemiology of Population Change. *Millbank Memorial Fund Quarterly* 49: 509–538.

IPCC. 2014. *Climate Change 2014: Synthesis Report.* Contribution of Working Groups I, II and III to the Fifth Assessment Report of the Intergovernmental Panel on Climate Change. Core Writing Team, Rajendra K. Pachauri and Leo A. Meyer, eds. IPCC, Geneva, Switzerland. https://www.ipcc.ch/report/ar5/syr/. Accessed 8 November 2022.

Rich, Paul. 1999. The Emergence and Significance of Warlordism in International Politics. In *Warlords in International Relations*, ed. Paul Rich, 1–16. New York: St. Martin's Press.

Sabatinelli, Guido. 2002. Determinants of Malaria in WHO European Region. In *The Contextual Determinants of Malaria*, ed. Elizabeth Casman and Hadi Dowlatabadi, 66–92. Washington, DC: Resources for the Future.

Schneider, Mary Jane. 2014. *Introduction to Public Health.* 4th ed. Burlington, MA: Jones and Barrett.

Shah, Sonia. 2010. *The Fever: How Malaria Has Ruled Mankind for 500,000 Years.* New York: Farrar, Straus and Giroux. Ibooks edition.

———. 2016. *Pandemic: Tracking Contagions from Cholera to Ebola and Beyond.* New York: Sarah Crichton Books.

Smith, Kirk R., Alistair Woodward, Diarmid Campbell-Lendrum, Dave D. Chadee, Yasushi Honda, Qiyong Liu, Jane M. Olwoch, Boris Revich, and Rainer Sauerborn. 2014. Human Health: Impacts, Adaptation, and Co-benefits. In *Climate Change 2014: Impacts, Adaptation, and Vulnerability. Part A: Global and Sectoral Aspects.* Contribution of Working Group II to the Fifth Assessment Report of the Intergovernmental Panel on Climate Change. Christopher B. Field, Vicente R. Barros, David J. Dokken, Katharine J. Mach, Michael D. Mastrandrea, T. Erin Bilir, Monalisa Chatterjee, Kristie L. Ebi, Yuka O. Estrada, Robert C. Genova, Betelhem Girma, Eric S. Kissel, Andrew N. Levy, Sandy MacCracken, Patricia R. Mastrandrea, and Leslie L. White, eds. https://www.ipcc.ch/report/ar5/syr/. Accessed 8 November 2022.

Sullivan, John. 2015. Sovereignty, Criminal Insurgency, and Drug Cartels: The Rise of a Post State Society. In *Warlords, Inc., Black Markets, Broken States and the Rise of the Warlord Entrepreneur*, ed. Noah Raford and Andrew Trabulsi, 95–119. Berkeley: North Atlantic Books. Apple Ibooks Edition.

Tishkov, Valery. 2004. *Chechnya: Life in a War-Torn Society.* Berkeley: University of California Press.

Trabulsi, Andrew. 2015. Warlords, Inc.-A Portrait. In *Warlords, Inc., Black Markets, Broken States and the Rise of the Warlord Entrepreneur*, ed. Noah Raford and Andrew Trabulsi, 27–46. Berkeley: North Atlantic Books.

UNECE. 2019. The State of Forests in the Caucasus and Central Asia. https://unece.org/DAM/timber/publications/sp-47-soccaf-en.pdf. Accessed 25 September 2022.

de Waal, Thomas. 2013. *Black Garden: Armenia and Azerbaijan Through Peace and War*. New York: New York University Press.
World Health Organization (WHO). 2019. *World Malaria Report*. Geneva: World Health Organization.
Zartman, William. 1995. Putting Things Back Together. In *Collapsed States: The Disintegration and Restoration of Legitimate Authority*, ed. William Zartman, 267–271. Boulder: Lynne Reinner.
Zurcher, Christopher. 2007. *The Post-Soviet Wars: Rebellion, Ethnic Conflict and Nationhood in the Caucasus*. New York: NYU Press.

# Appendix A: Research And Research Methods

## Archival Research

The first phase of this project involved a review of secondary literature to construct a basic timeline of the Karabakh conflict and the history of malaria in the Caucasus region. Key sources for the history of malaria included historic copies of *Public Health Reports* and other medical journals with epidemiological data detailing rates of malaria and other infectious diseases in the first half of the twentieth century. Key secondary sources for the history of the conflict period included excellent books by Laurence Broers (2021), Christopher Zurcher (2007), Thomas Goltz (1998) and Michael Croissant (1998) and the outstanding edited volume by Jan Koehler and Christopher Zurcher (2003). Newspaper archives were also consulted, including the *New York Times*, *Washington Post* and *Los Angeles Times*.

The review of secondary sources was followed by a research trip to the United States National Archives in College Park, Maryland to examine records from RG 90 (Records of the US Public Health Service) and RG 0286 (Records of the United States Agency for International Development). These included reports and correspondence from the League of Nations Malaria Commission in the 1930s as well as data from various malaria eradication programs in the United States. Archival materials from RG 0286 included diplomatic correspondence from USAID personnel working in Armenia in the aftermath of the 1988 earthquake and through the early



K. Hirschfeld et al., *New Wars and Old Plagues*,
https://doi.org/10.1007/978-3-031-31143-7

years of the Karabakh conflict. Many of these individuals were health professionals and their reports include detailed descriptions of Armenian health care facilities at the end of the Soviet period and during the transition.

These archival materials were incorporated into a detailed chronology of the conflict period further informed by conversations with a few key informants. These included Dr. Scott McNabb of the Centers for Disease Control who was an EIS (Epidemiology Intelligence Service) officer stationed in Armenia during the 1990s. We also spoke with Thomas Goltz, a journalist who reported extensively from Azerbaijan during the conflict. One of the goals of this historical timeline was to better contextualize the remote sensing data so the impact of the conflict could be assessed temporally and spatially. Some areas of the Karabakh region, for instance, endured repeated rounds of ethnic violence, depopulation and repopulation between 1988 and 1994. Other areas experienced fewer conflict events.

### *Site Visits to Armenia*

Our research was also informed by two site visits to Armenia. The first field excursion took place in June 2018 and the second took place in the winter of 2022. Both field visits were guided by Dr. Ani Melkonyan. During our 2018 visit we met and discussed our project with a number of different organizations. These included the Ministry of Emergency Situations National Hydrometerological Service, who provided helpful data on climatology and water resources. We also visited the Ministry of Nature Protection, the UNDP office, the Ministry of Health, the Ecocenter at the National Academy of Sciences Analytical Center for Risk Assessment, the Agrarian State University Department of Hydrotechnology, the American University in Armenia Department for Environmental Protection. The Minister of Agriculture arranged a visit to the Armavir region and connected us with a specialist from the Scientific Center of Agriculture and Plant Protection Experimental Farm. We were also given an opportunity to tour vineyards in the Argatsotn region. The German International Cooperation project office and faculty from Yerevan State University also contributed expertise.

Our 2022 visit to Armenia included visits to The National Center for Disease Control and Prevention in Yerevan where we met with the research group led by Dr. Lusine Paronyan. We discussed the current vector borne disease program and strategy for Armenia, including vector surveillance, mitigation, and abatement programs as well as the malaria case history following the WHO malaria free designation. At a second meeting with Dr. Paronyan's group, we had further discussions with Dr. Ara Keshishyan, former head of the Laboratory for Malaria within the Ministry of Health, on the historical case history of malaria and mitigation strategies in Soviet Armenia and the disease situation surrounding the first conflict in the early 1990s.

We also visited the Institute of Migration (IOM) within the United Nations complex in Yerevan. Our host was Nune Asatryan, Project Coordinator for IOM. She provided information on the status of migrants and refugees in Armenia, on the care and services surrounding those displaced in the fall 2020 conflict as well as historical information regarding the first conflict. IOM also provided web resources and other data on historical migrant and refugee reports.

The main research endeavor for our second site visit was a tour of the agricultural areas to south and west of Yerevan. This area was the center of the malaria outbreak in the mid to late 1990s following the first conflict with Azerbaijan. We spent two full days driving through rural agricultural villages in Armavir and Ararat provinces. At each village Dr. Melkonyan and Brad Brayfield interviewed individuals outside markets, homes, city centers and parks on their recollections of the past history of malaria during the conflict in the early 1990s as well as during Soviet times. Residents were also asked for recollections about any irrigation/water infrastructure projects implemented for mosquito mitigation and on their experience with mosquitos in their village. Visible irrigation infrastructure, agricultural crops, field status, fisheries and other infrastructure within these regions were explored and documented. Our team also drove to Gyumri, Vanadzor and along the Debed River in the north of Lori province, before returning to Yerevan. Here we documented the forest structure, forest lost, agricultural crops and practices. During our visit in between other activities, we conducted informal interviews with younger urban residents exploring issues of nationality and identity.

## *Spatial Data and Analysis*

### *Regional Borders and Geography*

Modern boundary shapefiles for national and subnational administrative units of the south Caucasus were obtained from GADM.org. The data was conflated to the Soviet Union shapefile to match boundaries. The state and regional boundaries for the former Soviet Union were derived from the 1:3 million scale administrative boundaries for the land area of the Former Soviet Union. This data was conflated with the 2020 ESRI country shapefile. Bodies of water and rivers were derived from ESRI World Water Hydropolys and/or Natural Earth. Open Street Map places area was used for cities and towns. Urban centers were obtained from Natural Earth.

*Conflict Region*

Mapping the conflict area, especially disputed territories, is difficult because clear border delineations are not readily available. For this project we first used the country borders and the Nagorno-Karabakh border from the ESRI country dataset. The Nagorno-Karabakh line of contact was downloaded from the website of the Armenian Ministry of Foreign Affairs (digitized on GitHub by https://github.com/mkudamatsu/data_karabakh-map). Next, to generate the newly renegotiated Nagorno-Karabakh boundary, we investigated an available UNHCR map (ACAPS 2020). In addition, we evaluated topographic maps in Google Earth to ensure the boundary was placed in accordance with topographic relief and the location of urban areas. For example, we placed the new line with attention to several of the areas which were known to have turned over in the conflict, such as Mataghis dam in the north, Agdam district in the east and Shusha City in the south. Additionally, we corroborated this update by examining maps produced by the Russian Ministry of Defense peacekeeping forces (Russian Ministry of Defence 2020). The boundary created in this manner is not an official boundary and only represents an approximation of the fully negotiated boundary.

*Conflict Sites*

Conflict site data from the Nagorno-Karabakh conflict between Armenia and Azerbaijan was obtained from the Peace Research Institute Oslo (PRIO) website https://ucdp.uu.se/downloads/). These data were compiled and maintained through a collaboration between the Department of Peace and Conflict Research at Uppsala University and the Centre for the Study of Civil War at PRIO (https://www.pcr.uu.se/research/ucdp/methodology/). These datasets have been widely used for conflict research for many years. These events are compiled by human coders that mine global news sources, NGO reports, case studies, truth commission reports, historical archives and other sources of information using computer search. Subsequently, all collected events were analyzed for accuracy and redundancy. All data concerning the event, including the actors involved, location of the conflict event, and the number of deaths is retrieved and stored. Geolocated conflict events for Fig. 3.1 were obtained from the UCDP Georeferenced Event Dataset (GED) Global version 22.1 which is composed of events from 1989 through 2021 (Sundberg and Melander 2013). The newest GED datasets compile events involving armed organized actors against other organized actors or civilian groups which resulted in at least one estimated fatality. Thus, events include those pertaining to state, non-state and one-sided based actors and/or civilians. All events specific to Armenia, Nagorno-Karabakh or Azerbaijan occurring between 1989 and 2020 which had known precise locations (city/town/village) or within 25km of specific locations were selected and analyzed in ArcMap 10.7. Events with location precision only at the district, rayon or national level were excluded from analysis in Fig. 3.1. Death counts for conflict events used in Fig. 3.1B were based on the "best" estimate of deaths variable, and only precise events of the same criteria detailed above were considered.

*UNHCR Refugee and IDP Settlement Camps*

The settlement sites which housed IDP and refugees in Armenia and Azerbaijan were selected from the global United Nations High Commission for Refugees georeferenced settlement dataset, (https://gis.unhcr.org/arcgis/rest/services/core/wrl_ppl_poc_p_unhcr/FeatureServer). The shapefile with global data was uploaded as a layer, projection set and camps within Armenia and Azerbaijan were selected by location attributes as completely within the boundary. Layers highlighting active camps (as of 2019) and previous camps were generated.

*Irrigated Cropland Estimates*

The percentage of irrigation croplands for south Caucasus region was determined by analyzing the Copernicus Global Land Service dataset at 100 × 100m. This dataset was adapted to find irrigated croplands based on MODIS Land surface temperature maximums (summer 2015) and Landsat NDVI (summer average from 2015). The percent cropland analysis was based on data from 2015 and 2019. As a result, it may not accurately reflect the actual amount of irrigation that was occurring in these locations prior and during the time of conflict. Further work on a much finer spatial scale and over a time series would add significantly to the data analysis.

*Census Data and Human Mobility*
Census numbers of NGK and Azerbaijan were obtained and confirmed authentic as above from the websites http://www.ethno-kavkaz.narod.ru/rnkarabax.html and http://www.ethno-kavkaz.narod.ru/rnazerbaijan.html. This site contains tables compiled from official statistics of the Central Statistics Administration of the Soviet Union.

For the human mobility analysis, population data was obtained from primary and secondary published sources online. Census data on the Nagorno-Karabakh region was obtained from the website of the National Statistical Service of the Republic of Artsakh (http://www.stat-nkr.am/en). The census information from the 2005 and 2015 official census, as well as a summary of the ethnic composition of Nagorno-Karabakh region is included in the 2005 census results. Online documents deemed reliable by Dr. Melkonyan were translated into English. Overall, it is estimated that approximately a million people (both Armenian and Azerbaijani) were displaced from NGK and neighboring rayons because of the conflict, with the vast majority being Azerbaijani (UNHCR 2009). Data on involvement of foreign fighters during the conflict is limited.

*Malaria*
Cases of malaria in Armenia were compiled from published reports from the World Health Organization World Malaria Report 1982–2010. This data was supplemented with published research reports summarizing the cases of malaria in Armenia, Azerbaijan, Georgia and Tajikistan. Cases of malaria by province were merged with shapefiles of subnational boundaries as detailed above within ArcMap project layers.

*Integration of Qualitative Research with Remote Sensing Data*
Our research group met bi-weekly for discussions and updates between 2018 and 2021. During these meetings we shared our respective findings and looked for opportunities to apply advances in one segment of the research to better contextualize data and information obtained from other segments. The construction of a formal historical timeline informed by primary source material, for instance, helped better frame the analysis of

remote sensing data to assess the impact of specific phases of the conflict on the natural environment. We were also fortunate to have Dr. Ani Melkonyan in residence at the University of Oklahoma during the 2019–2020 academic year to provide additional insight and contacts from her extensive professional network in Armenia. Our site visits allowed us to document the physical landscape of the Armenian countryside and these visuals further informed our geospatial data analysis. Site visits also provided a more human perspective as individual Armenian families and researchers volunteered their recollections of the hardships they experienced during the conflict in the 1990s.

## References

ACAPS: https://www.acaps.org/. Accessed 2020.

Russian Ministry of Defence of the Russian Federation: Russian peacekeeping forces in Nagorno-Karabakh. Accessed 2020. https://eng.mil.ru/en/russian_peacekeeping_forces/infographics.htm.

UNHCR Report. 2009. *Azerbaijan: Analysis of Gaps in the Protection of Internally Displaced Persons (IDPs)*. UN High Commission for Refugees (UNHCR).

# Appendix B: Historical Chronology of the Conflict

## Pre Soviet Era, 1915–1921

1915–1922 Armenian genocide

1917 Bolsheviks seize power in Russia

1918 Republic of Azerbaijan founded

1918 Republic of Armenia founded

1921 Famine and epidemic malaria reported across the southern Caucasus and Russia

## Soviet Era 1921–1990

1918–1921 South Caucasus incorporated into USSR, but Karabakh region remains independent

1921 June Caucasus bureau of the CCP took up the question of Karabakh and declared it part of Armenia. Stalin allegedly engineered a reversal the next day and Karabakh was declared part of Azerbaijan SSR with Shusha the administrative center

1922 December USSR creates new composite Transcaucasus Soviet Federative Socialist Republic and annexes all Caucasus republics as a single entity

1923 Karabakh becomes reclassified as an AO (Autonomous Oblast) within the territory of Azerbaijan

1924 Lenin dies, Stalin ascends to power

1933 United States formally recognizes USSR


K. Hirschfeld et al., *New Wars and Old Plagues*,
https://doi.org/10.1007/978-3-031-31143-7

1934 USSR joins League of Nations

1936 New Soviet constitution. Azeri Turks and Turkic language reclassified as Azerbaijani

1937–1947 Stalinist purges throughout Caucasus. Mass deportations of entire ethnic groups

1953 Stalin dies. Khrushchev in power

1963 Malaria declared eradicated in Armenia

## Late Soviet Period, 1987–1990

1987 October Azeri officials in Karabakh transfer land from an Armenian collective farm (Kolkhoz) to Azeri Kolkhoz, leading to protests and riots by Armenians. Soviet authorities responded aggressively to contain protests, leading to multiple demonstrations in Armenian cities and towns

1987 November outbreaks of violence in Karabakh. Referendum petition sent to Soviet Premier Gorbachev

1988 February vote by Karabakh Committee to leave Azerbaijan. Violent pogroms in Azeri city of Sumgait. Over 180,000 Armenians flee Azerbaijan for Armenia

1988 June Azeri supreme Soviet passes resolution affirming Karabakh is part of Azerbaijan

1988 September Armenians expelled from Karabakh town of Shusha. Azeris expelled from villages and rural areas in Karabakh. Expulsions intensify and hundreds of thousands forced to relocate

1988 December Armenian earthquake. 25000 killed. Over 100,000 people homeless

1989 Ethnic militias intensify violence in Karabakh. Hundreds of thousands forced to relocate

1990 "Black January" Anti-Armenian pogrom in Baku. Soviet troops kill over 100 demonstrators. Karabakh placed under direct rule by Moscow

1990 Almost all Soviet SSRs and ASSRs declare independence and assert sovereignty

1990–1991 Operation Ring. Soviet and Azeri troops encircle Armenian villages in Karabakh in an attempt to disarm separatist militias. Many atrocities reported

1991 August Azerbaijan declares independence from USSR

1991 September coup attempt in Moscow collapses

1991 September Armenia declares independence from USSR

1991 September 1991 New republic of Nagorno-Karabakh created with capital city of Stepanakert

1991 November Azerbaijan shuts down gas pipeline into Armenia creating severe energy crisis

1991 December Soviet military gear appropriated by ethnic militias. Conflict intensifies

## Post-Soviet Era, 1992–Present

1992–1993 conflict intensifies. Many villages in Karabakh depopulated and repopulated several times

1992 May Peace talks in Tashkent. Soviet arms stores divided among successor nations

1992 May Armenians create Lachin corridor, a land bridge linking Karabakh with Armenia

1992 September Peace talks in Sochi fail to diminish conflict

1992 September–October Massive offshore oil and gas reserves discovered in Azerbaijan. Azerbaijani military offensive regains territory around Karabakh

1992 December USAID sends additional humanitarian relief to Armenia, including team of epidemiologists from US Centers for Disease Control

1993 spring Armenian offensive captures significant territory outside of Karabakh

1993 May Aliyev returns to power in Azerbaijan, attempts to consolidate power over warlords and unify military

1994 May cease fire negotiated in Bishkek Kyrgyzstan. Karabakh conflict becomes "frozen." Malaria epidemic recognized in Armenia and control measures implemented

1994 October Azerbaijan signs $7 billion deal for oil exploration

1998 World Health Organization begins "Roll Back Malaria" campaign

2000–2020 Ongoing low intensity violence in Karabakh

2020 Major escalation of conflict resolves with peace accord transferring land controlled by Armenia to Azerbaijan

2022 Sporadic outbreaks of violence and public protests in Armenia against proposed transfer of land

# Index




K. Hirschfeld et al., *New Wars and Old Plagues*,
https://doi.org/10.1007/978-3-031-31143-7

CPSIA information can be obtained
at www.ICGtesting.com
Printed in the USA
LVHW081129150623
749849LV00001B/3

9 783031 311420